# REPORT DOCUMENTATION PAGE

| 1. AGENCY USE ONLY (Leave blank) | 2. REPORT DATE<br>September 2005 | 3. REPORT TYPE AND DATES COVERED<br>Final Report<br>January 2003–December 2003 |
|---|---|---|

**4. TITLE AND SUBTITLE**
Drug and Alcohol Testing Results 2003 Annual Report

**5. FUNDING NUMBERS**
TMB8/BB241

**6. AUTHOR(S)**
Randy Clarke*, Robert Gaumer*, Michael Redington, and Eve Rutyna

**7. PERFORMING ORGANIZATION NAME(S) AND ADDRESS(ES)**
U.S. Department of Transportation
Research and Innovative Technology Administration
John A. Volpe National Transportation Systems Center
55 Broadway
Cambridge, MA 02142-1093

**8. PERFORMING ORGANIZATION REPORT NUMBER**
DOT-VNTSC-FTA-05-06

**9. SPONSORING/MONITORING AGENCY NAME(S) AND ADDRESS(ES)**
U.S. Department of Transportation
Federal Transit Administration
Office of Safety and Security
Washington, DC 20590

**10. SPONSORING/MONITORING AGENCY REPORT NUMBER**
FTA-MA-26-0054-06-1

**11. SUPPLEMENTARY NOTES**
*Chenega Advanced Solutions and Engineering (CASE).
55 Broadway
Cambridge, MA 02142-1093

**12a. DISTRIBUTION/AVAILABILITY STATEMENT**
This document is available to the public through the National Technical Information Service, Springfield, VA 22161

**12b. DISTRIBUTION CODE**

**13. ABSTRACT (Maximum 200 words)**

This is the eighth annual report of the results of the Federal Transit Administration's (FTA) Drug and Alcohol Testing Program. The report summarizes the new reporting requirements introduced for calendar year 2003, the requirements of the overall drug and alcohol testing program (the revised CFR Part 40 and CFR Part 655), the results from the data reported for 2003, and the random drug and alcohol violation rates (the percentage of persons selected for a random test who produced a positive specimen or refused to take the test) for calendar years 1996 through 2003.

The results of drug tests—for marijuana, cocaine, phencyclidine (PCP), opiates, and amphetamines—are compared with the results of alcohol tests for the various types of required tests. Statistics are presented for random, post-accident, reasonable suspicion, and pre-employment tests combined and for each individual test type. Those test results are further compared by employer type (transit agencies and contractors), employer size (large, small, and rural), employee category, FTA region, and the drug type.

Statistics on employees returned to duty and results of return to duty tests and follow-up tests are presented separately from results of the other four test types because return-to-duty tests and follow-up tests represent a different segment of the test population and not all employers offer rehabilitation.

**14. SUBJECT TERMS**
alcohol testing, drug testing, random testing, safety-sensitive, return to duty, rates

**15. NUMBER OF PAGES**
84

**16. PRICE CODE**

| 17. SECURITY CLASSIFICATION OF REPORT<br>Unclassified | 18. SECURITY CLASSIFICATION OF THIS PAGE<br>Unclassified | 19. SECURITY CLASSIFICATION OF THIS ABSTRACT<br>Unclassified | 20. LIMITATION OF ABSTRACT<br>Unlimited |
|---|---|---|---|

# Preface

This annual report represents the cooperative efforts of many people. Extensive appreciation is extended to the U.S. Department of Transportation's Federal Transit Administration, the Volpe National Transportation Systems Center, and the following individuals who were instrumental in guiding this project and contributing to its success:

Michael Taborn
Director, Office of Transit Safety and Security
Federal Transit Administration

Jerry Powers
Drug and Alcohol Program Manager
Federal Transit Administration

Michael R. Redington
Program Manager/Transportation Industry Analyst
Volpe National Transportation Systems Center

# METRIC/ENGLISH CONVERSION FACTORS

## ENGLISH TO METRIC

### LENGTH (APPROXIMATE)

1 inch (in) = 2.5 centimeters (cm)

1 foot (ft) = 30 centimeters (cm)

1 yard (yd) = 0.9 meter (m)

1 mile (mi) = 1.6 kilometers (km)

### AREA (APPROXIMATE)

1 square inch (sq in, $in^2$) = 6.5 square centimeters ($cm^2$)

1 square foot (sq ft, $ft^2$) = 0.09 square meter ($m^2$)

1 square yard (sq yd, $yd^2$) = 0.8 square meter ($m^2$)

1 square mile (sq mi, $mi^2$) = 2.6 square kilometers ($km^2$)

1 acre = 0.4 hectare (he) = 4,000 square meters ($m^2$)

### MASS - WEIGHT (APPROXIMATE)

1 ounce (oz) = 28 grams (gm)

1 pound (lb) = 0.45 kilogram (kg)

1 short ton = 2,000 pounds (lb) = 0.9 tonne (t)

### VOLUME (APPROXIMATE)

1 teaspoon (tsp) = 5 milliliters (ml)

1 tablespoon (tbsp) = 15 milliliters (ml)

1 fluid ounce (fl oz) = 30 milliliters (ml)

1 cup (c) = 0.24 liter (l)

1 pint (pt) = 0.47 liter (l)

1 quart (qt) = 0.96 liter (l)

1 gallon (gal) = 3.8 liters (l)

1 cubic foot (cu ft, $ft^3$) = 0.03 cubic meter ($m^3$)

1 cubic yard (cu yd, $yd^3$) = 0.76 cubic meter ($m^3$)

### TEMPERATURE (EXACT)

$[(x-32)(5/9)]$ °F = y °C

## METRIC TO ENGLISH

### LENGTH (APPROXIMATE)

1 millimeter (mm) = 0.04 inch (in)

1 centimeter (cm) = 0.4 inch (in)

1 meter (m) = 3.3 feet (ft)

1 meter (m) = 1.1 yards (yd)

1 kilometer (km) = 0.6 mile (mi)

### AREA (APPROXIMATE)

1 square centimeter ($cm^2$) = 0.16 square inch (sq in, $in^2$)

1 square meter ($m^2$) = 1.2 square yards (sq yd, $yd^2$)

1 square kilometer ($km^2$) = 0.4 square mile (sq mi, $mi^2$)

10,000 square meters ($m^2$) = 1 hectare (ha) = 2.5 acres

### MASS - WEIGHT (APPROXIMATE)

1 gram (gm) = 0.036 ounce (oz)

1 kilogram (kg) = 2.2 pounds (lb)

1 tonne (t) = 1,000 kilograms (kg)

= 1.1 short tons

### VOLUME (APPROXIMATE)

1 milliliter (ml) = 0.03 fluid ounce (fl oz)

1 liter (l) = 2.1 pints (pt)

1 liter (l) = 1.06 quarts (qt)

1 liter (l) = 0.26 gallon (gal)

1 cubic meter ($m^3$) = 36 cubic feet (cu ft, $ft^3$)

1 cubic meter ($m^3$) = 1.3 cubic yards (cu yd, $yd^3$)

### TEMPERATURE (EXACT)

$[(9/5) y + 32]$ °C = x °F

## QUICK INCH - CENTIMETER LENGTH CONVERSION

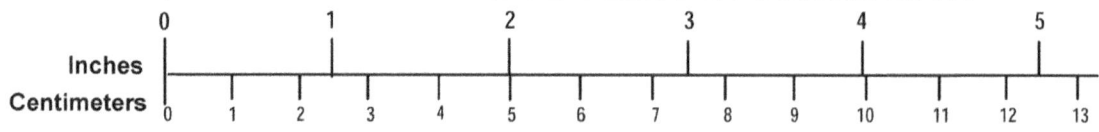

## QUICK FAHRENHEIT - CELSIUS TEMPERATURE CONVERSION

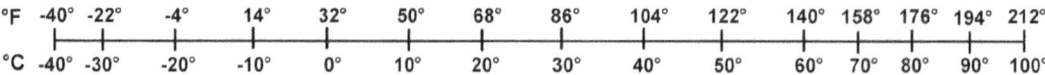

For more exact and or other conversion factors, see NIST Miscellaneous Publication 286, Units of Weights and Measures. Price $2.50 SD Catalog No. C13 10286

Updated 6/17/98

# Executive Summary

Federal Transit Administration (FTA) regulations require that each recipient (both direct and indirect) of FTA funds (1) implement an anti-drug program to deter and detect the use of prohibited drugs, (2) establish a program to prevent the misuse of alcohol, and (3) report the results of its programs to FTA upon request. Compliance with FTA's drug and alcohol testing program is a condition of federal assistance. Failure of a recipient to establish and implement a drug and alcohol testing program – either in its own operations or in those of an entity operating on its behalf – may result in the suspension of FTA funding to the recipient.

Employees who perform any of five safety-sensitive functions must be tested for five controlled substances[1] in four circumstances: random, post-accident, reasonable suspicion, and pre-employment. Such employees must also be tested for alcohol use in each of those circumstances except pre-employment, though employers may, and many do, require pre-employment tests per 49CFR Part 40 testing procedures. An additional circumstance (return to duty/follow-up) is required for safety-sensitive employees who are given an opportunity to resume safety-sensitive duties after testing positive for drugs or alcohol or refusing to submit to a required test.

## Random Rates

FTA considers random testing to be the most effective deterrent to drug use and alcohol misuse. The results of random tests also provide the best indication of the overall level of drug use and alcohol misuse, and the combined percentage of positive random tests plus random test refusals are used by FTA in determining minimum random testing rates for the following year. The test result rates for drugs and alcohol, respectively, that are used in determining the testing rates for the following year are calculated as follows:

*(verified drug positives + refusals) ÷ (total number of testing events[2])*

*(confirmed alcohol positives[3] + refusals) ÷ (total number of testing events)*

In 2003, 1,170 verified random drug test positives and 129 random drug test refusals were reported. Additionally, 37 random alcohol tests were reported with a confirmed blood alcohol level of at least .04, and 11 refusals to take a random alcohol test were reported.

---

[1] The five substances that must be tested for are marijuana, cocaine, phencyclidine (PCP), opiates, and amphetamines.

[2] Per the addition of Section 26 and Appendix H to Part 40 in 2003, a testing event includes test refusals but not canceled tests.

[3] A positive alcohol test is a confirmation screen with a breath alcohol level of at least 0.04.

## Official Random Rates for 2003

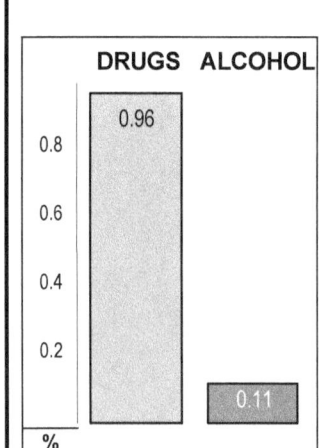

The graph at left shows the "official" rates for random drug and random alcohol tests used by the FTA Administrator in determining future random testing rates.

Because the random drug rate must remain below 1.0 percent for two consecutive years before it can be lowered and the rate in 2002 was above 1.0 percent, the random testing rate for drugs remained at 50 percent for 2004. If the rate remains below 1.0 percent in 2004, the FTA Administrator will have the option to reduce the random drug test quota for 2005 to 25 percent.

Because the 2003 alcohol rate was below 0.50 percent, the random testing quota for alcohol remained at 10 percent for 2004.

## Rates for Four Types of Testing

The combined percentages of positive tests plus test refusals shown in the previous graph are compared with the same rates for post-accident, reasonable suspicion, and pre-employment tests and for the four test types combined, in the graph at right. The rates for return to duty and follow-up tests are presented in a separate graph because those tests represent a different segment of the test population (i.e., tests produced by persons who have been removed from duty for drug or alcohol violations and have completed a rehabilitation program) and not all employers offer rehabilitation.

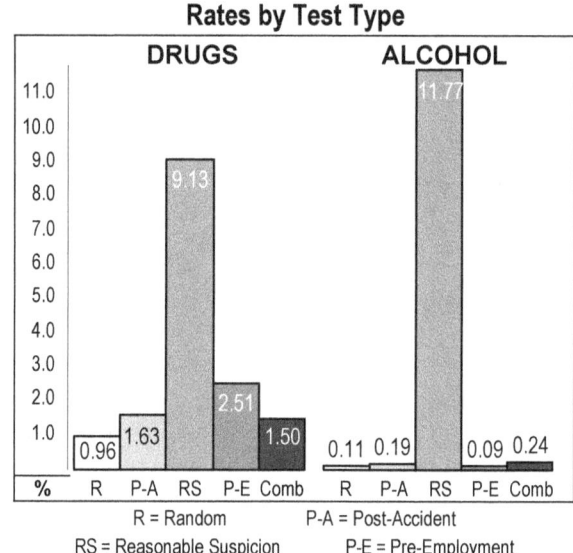

As shown, the reasonable suspicion rates were much higher than the random, post-accident, or pre-employment rates for both drugs and alcohol. The random rate was the lowest of the drug rates, significantly lower than the positive rates for any of the other three test types. The pre-employment rate was the lowest of the alcohol rates, and the random rate was slightly higher.

There were 135,297 random drug testing events reported in 2003, and 215,443 were reported for the four test types combined. The fewest reported were for reasonable suspicion, at 657. Next was post-accident, at 13,715. There were 42,317 random alcohol testing events reported in 2003, and 65,099 were reported for the four test types combined. The fewest reported were for reasonable suspicion, at 620. Next was post-accident, at 12,490. Only 9,672 pre-employment alcohol testing events were reported compared with 65,774 for drugs, reflecting the fact that pre-employment drug testing is required and pre-employment alcohol testing is not required

## Employer Type and Size

As shown in the following two graphs, the rates for contractors were higher than those for transit agency employees for each test type for drugs and for each test type for alcohol except random, which was slightly higher for transit employees. The random drug rate was more than twice as high for contractors. The combined alcohol rate was also nearly twice as high for contractors, and the combined drug rate was more than two-and-one-half times as high for contractors. Many more testing events were reported for transit agency employees than for contractors for both drugs and alcohol—three to four times as many for each test type except pre-employment events, twice as many for pre-employment alcohol tests and one-third more for pre-employment drug tests.

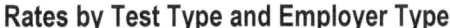

**Rates by Test Type and Employer Type**

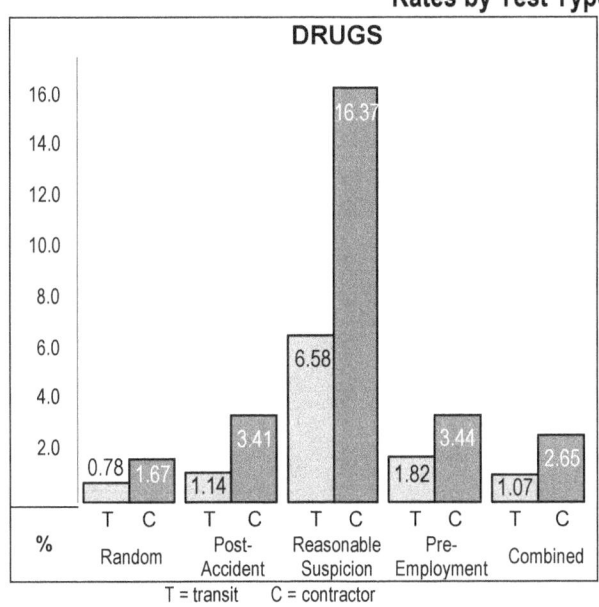
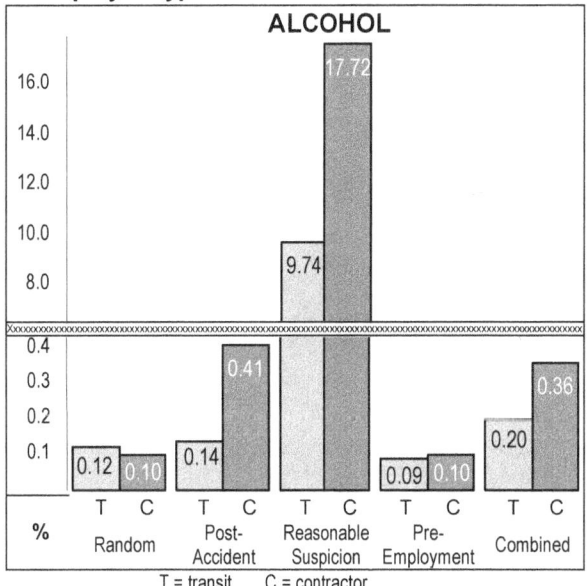

As shown in the next two graphs, the rates for the three employer size categories were very similar for the four types combined for both drugs and alcohol. The greatest variation in both the drug and alcohol rates by employer size was for reasonable suspicion, and large employers reported the lowest rates for both. Small employers reported the highest random drug rates, and rural employers reported the highest random alcohol rates. More than 80 percent of the testing events reported for both drugs and alcohol were reported by large employers. Rural employers reported approximately twice as many random testing events as small employers for both drugs and alcohol. That ratio of testing events is approximately the same for all four test types combined.

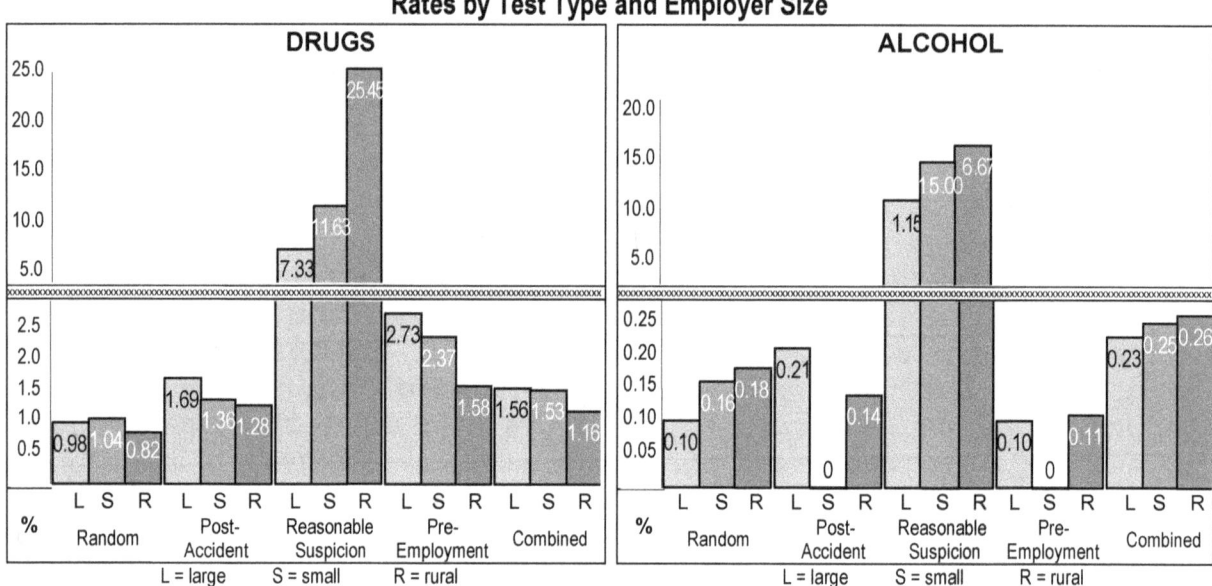

### Employee Category

The armed security personnel category had the lowest drug rate for all test types and the lowest alcohol rate for all test types except random. The

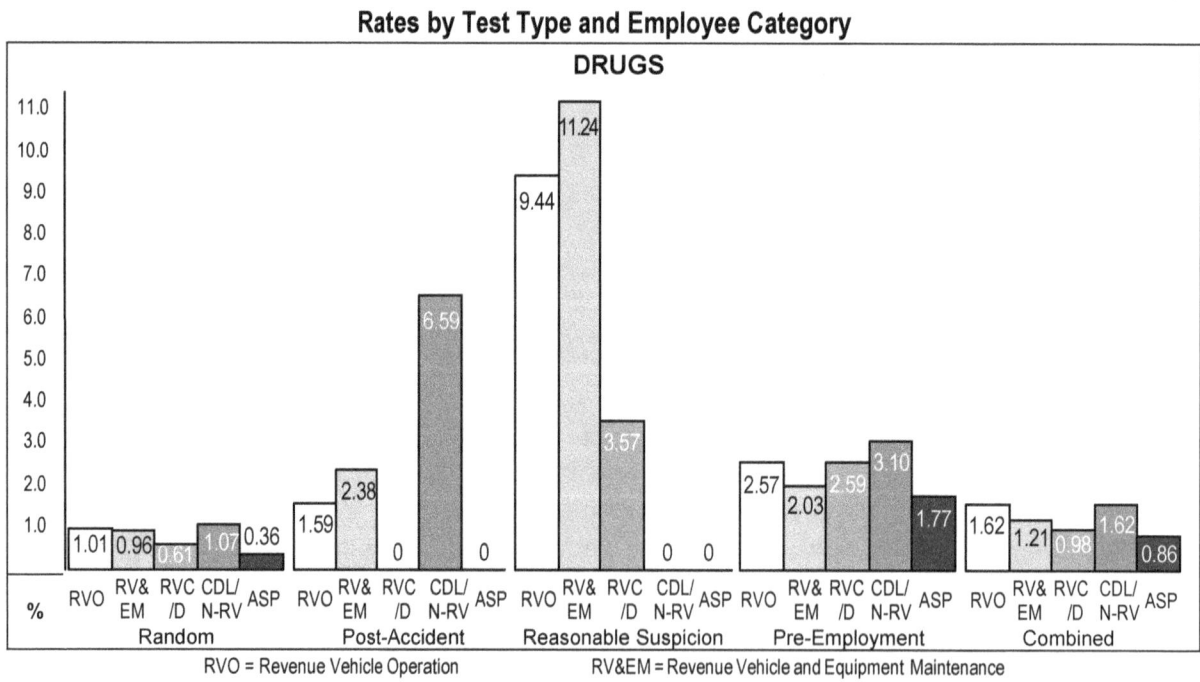

## Rates by Test Type and Employee Category

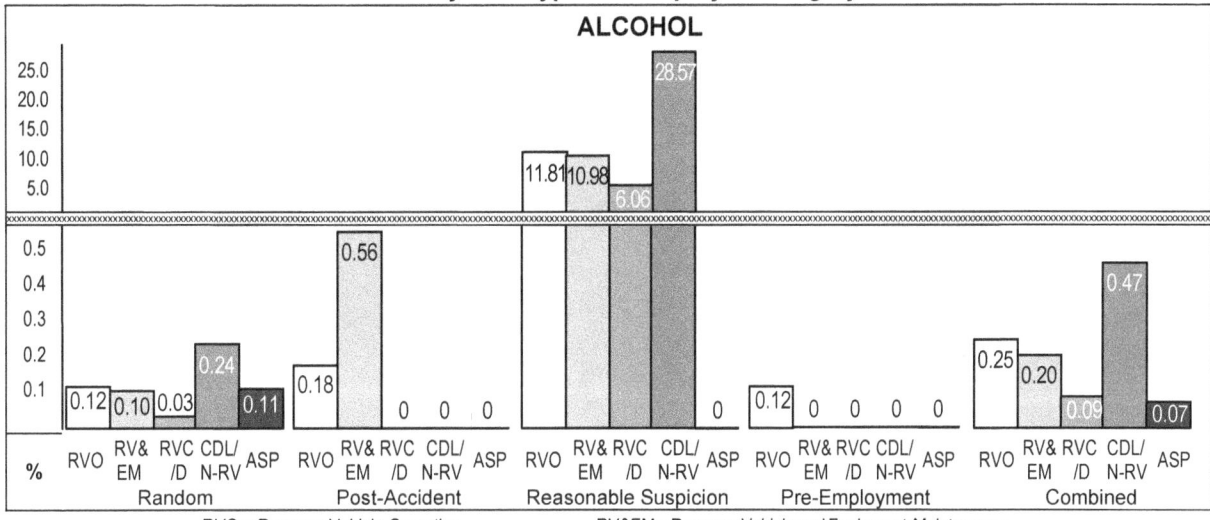

### ALCOHOL

RVO = Revenue Vehicle Operation    RV&EM = Revenue Vehicle and Equipment Maintenance
RVC/D = Revenue Vehicle Control/Dispatching    CDL/N-RV = CDL/Non-Revenue Vehicle    ASP = Armed Security Personnel

CDL[4]/non-revenue vehicle category had the highest drug rate for all test types except reasonable suspicion, the highest random alcohol rate, and the highest combined rate for alcohol. The vast majority of testing events reported for both drugs and alcohol were for the revenue vehicle operation category— approximately 70 percent of random tests, more than 80 percent of pre-employment and reasonable suspicion tests, and nearly 95 percent of post-accident tests. The revenue vehicle and equipment maintenance category had the second largest number of reported testing events for each test type for both drugs and alcohol.

### FTA Region

As shown on the map at right, the random drug rate was lowest in Region 2 at 0.63 percent, and was highest in Region 8 at 1.42 percent. Half of the regions had rates lower than the national average of 0.96 percent. The other half were more than 1.0 percent.

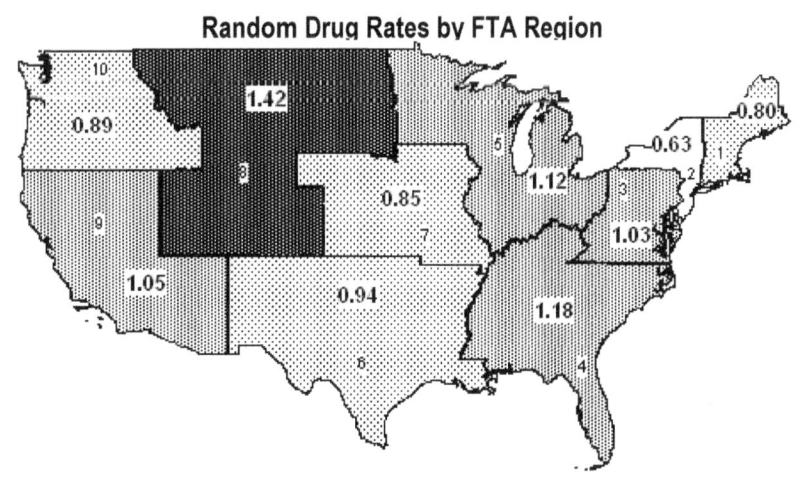

Random Drug Rates by FTA Region

---

[4] CDL = commercial driver license

As shown on the map at right, the random alcohol rate was zero in Region 8 and was by far the highest in Region 7 at 0.49 percent. Half of the regions had rates higher than the national average of 0.11 percent. All but Region 7 were less than 0.20 percent.

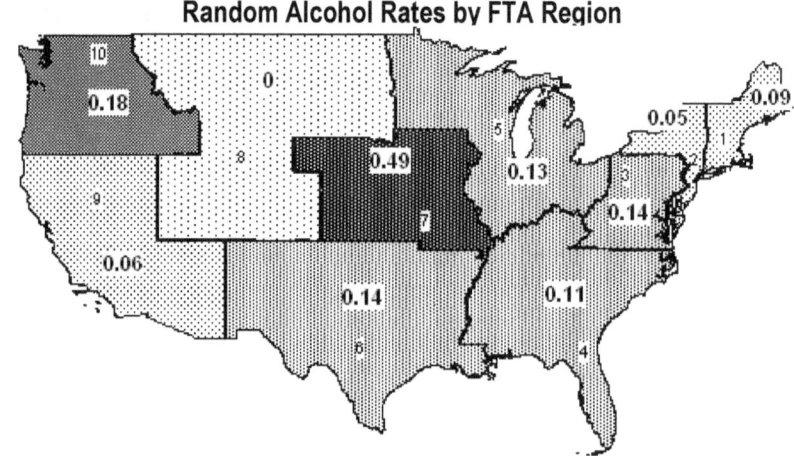

**Random Alcohol Rates by FTA Region**

### Type of Drug

As shown in the following charts, marijuana was detected more often than all of the other drugs combined in random testing, post-accident testing, pre-employment testing, and all four test types combined. Cocaine was detected most often in reasonable suspicion tests, and marijuana was second.

**Percentage by Drug Type of Total Drug Detections for Each Test Type**

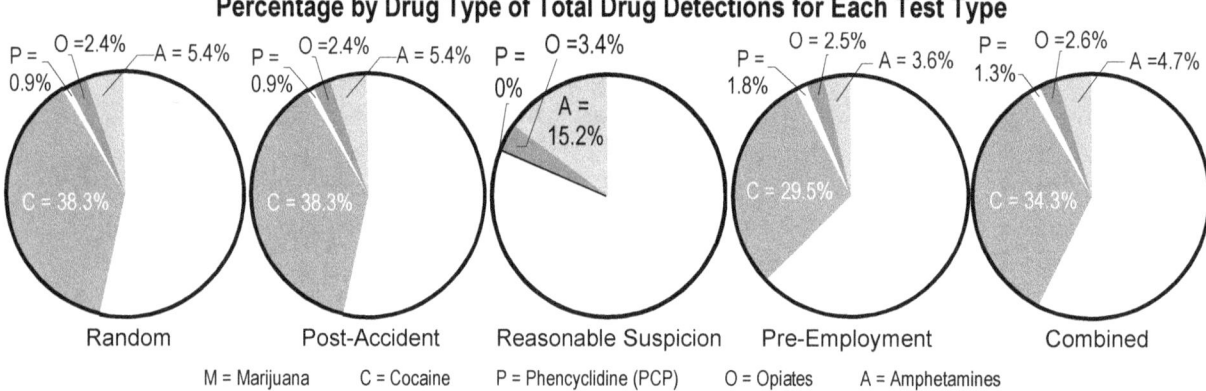

Random    Post-Accident    Reasonable Suspicion    Pre-Employment    Combined

M = Marijuana    C = Cocaine    P = Phencyclidine (PCP)    O = Opiates    A = Amphetamines

## Rates for Return to Duty Testing and Follow-Up Testing

Before being returned to duty, employees must complete a rehabilitation program and submit either a negative drug specimen or a negative alcohol screen, depending on the test that the employee initially failed or refused to take.

In 2003, 1,283 return to duty drug testing events, 713 return to duty alcohol testing events, 7,980 follow-up drug testing events, and 5,950 follow-up alcohol testing events were reported. Only three positive return to duty alcohol tests and one refusal were reported. Only 17 positive follow-up alcohol tests and two refusals were reported. As shown in the graphs at right, the return to

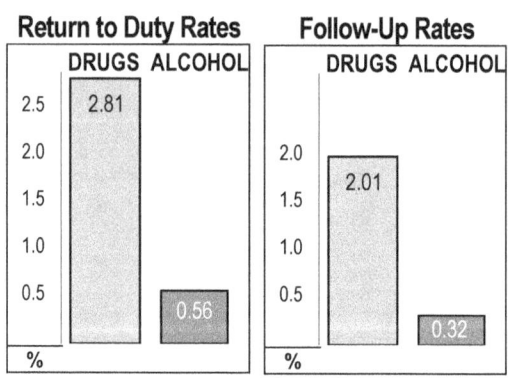

duty rates were higher than follow-up rates for both drugs and alcohol, and the alcohol rates were much lower than the drug rates.

Approximately 80 percent of the return to duty drug testing events were reported by transit agencies, and approximately 90 percent of return to duty alcohol testing events were reported by transit agencies. As shown in the graph at near right below, both the return to duty drug and alcohol rates for transit employees were higher than those for contractors. No positive alcohol tests or refusals were reported by contractors. More than 80 percent of the return to duty testing events were reported by large employers, and more than 90 percent of the alcohol testing events were reported by large employers. As shown in the graph at far right (above, the return to duty drug rate was much higher for large employers than that for small or rural employers, and no positive alcohol tests or refusals were reported by small or rural employers.

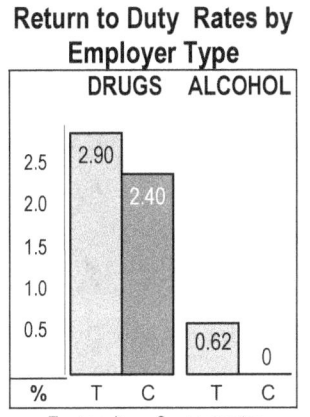

Return to Duty Rates by Employer Type

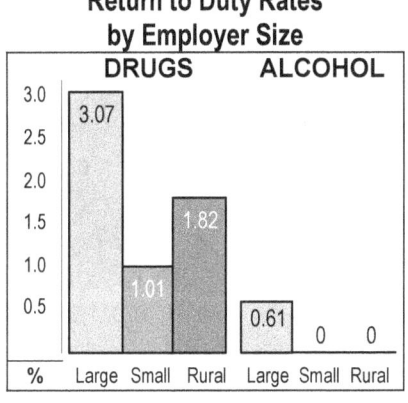

Return to Duty Rates by Employer Size

Approximately 90 percent of the follow-up testing events for both drugs and alcohol were reported by transit agencies. As shown in the graph at near right, the follow-up drug rates for contractors were twice as high as thosc for transit employees while the alcohol rate for transit agency employees was nearly twice as high as that for contractors. Nearly 95 percent of the follow-up drug testing events were reported by large employers, and nearly 98 percent of the follow-up alcohol testing events were reported by large employers. As shown in the graph at far right on the previous page, both the follow-up drug and alcohol rates for large employers were much lower than those for small or rural employers, and both rates for small and rural were similar. Despite the

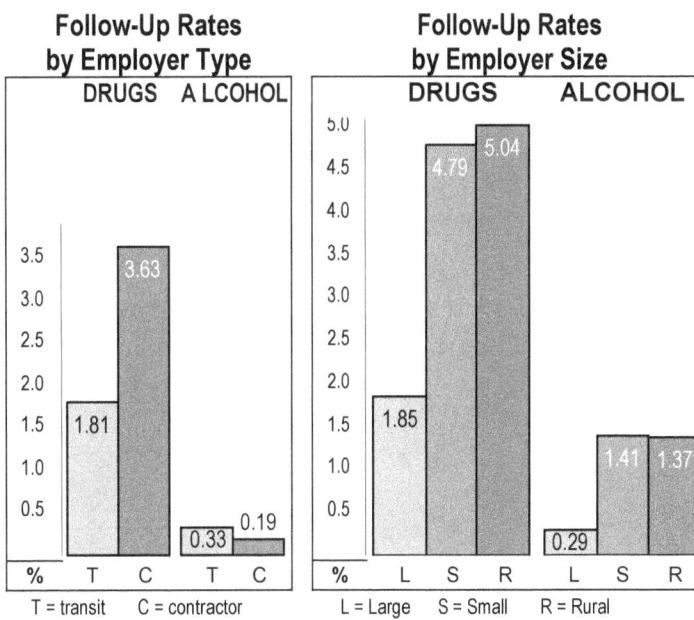

relatively high rates, only one positive alcohol test and no refusals were reported by both small and rural employers.

## Trends: 1996 through 2003

In 2001, FTA eliminated its requirement that all direct recipients report data each year, and developed a random sampling technique to select a portion of the recipients to report their data. Therefore, the only rates that can be reliably compared for each year of reporting (from 1996 to 2003) are random rates. The results actually reported in 2001 and 2002 do not accurately reflect total FTA testing due to the large proportion of results reported by large employers. Thus, the results from random testing were weighted to obtain "official" random rates that reasonably estimate the rate for all persons tested, enabling reliable comparison with the years before 2001 when all employers were required to report. Weighted rates are not available for any test types other than random or any subsets of random testing.

As shown in the following graph, the official random drug rate dropped in 2003 to the lowest rate (0.96 percent) since employers in all size categories were required to report, following its only rise (in 2002). The 2003 rate was 40 percent lower than the rate in 1996. As also shown in the next graph, the official random alcohol rate dropped by 50 percent in 2003 to 0.11 percent, by far the lowest rate since employers in all size categories were required to report.

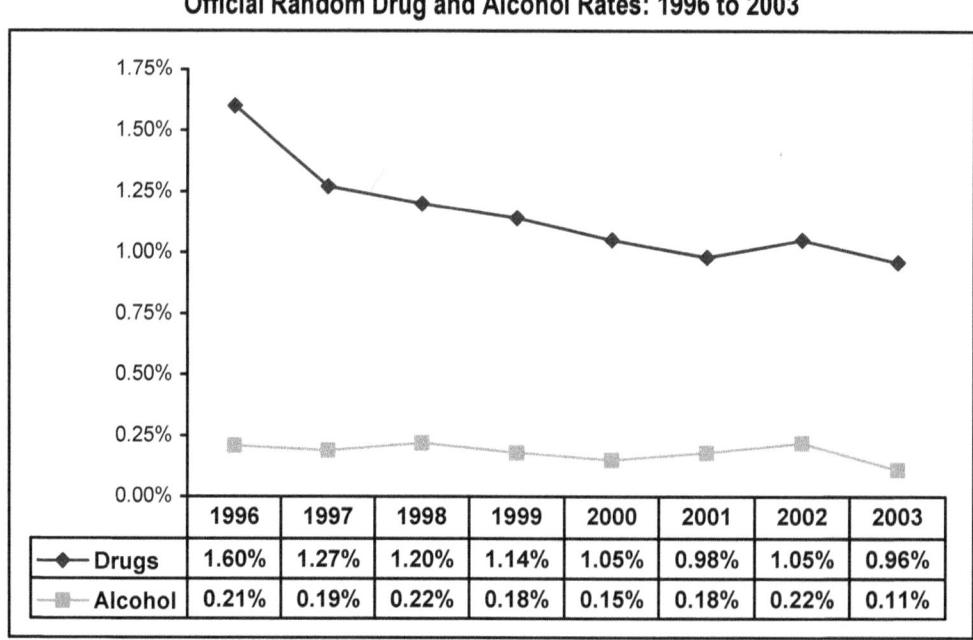

**Official Random Drug and Alcohol Rates: 1996 to 2003**

|         | 1996  | 1997  | 1998  | 1999  | 2000  | 2001  | 2002  | 2003  |
|---------|-------|-------|-------|-------|-------|-------|-------|-------|
| Drugs   | 1.60% | 1.27% | 1.20% | 1.14% | 1.05% | 0.98% | 1.05% | 0.96% |
| Alcohol | 0.21% | 0.19% | 0.22% | 0.18% | 0.15% | 0.18% | 0.22% | 0.11% |

# Table of Contents

# 1. Introduction

This report is the eighth annual summary of data submitted for entry in the Federal Transit Administration's (FTA) Drug and Alcohol Management Information System (DAMIS). The report summarizes data reported for calendar year 2003, and includes a comparison of official random drug and alcohol test rates for calendar years 1996 through 2003. DAMIS contains the data from all the drug and alcohol tests conducted under FTA regulations between 1996 and 2000, but contains data from only selected agencies for the years since 2000, as explained in Section 1.2. DAMIS also contains the data from all the tests conducted by large agencies in 1995.

FTA regulations require recipients and subrecipients of funding under Title 49 of United States Code (U.S.C.) Sections 5307, 5309, and 5311, and 23 U.S.C. Section 103(e)(4) and their contractors to implement and maintain a program to deter and detect use of prohibited drugs and misuse of alcohol by safety-sensitive employees, unless the recipient is also an operating railroad regulated by the Federal Railroad Administration (FRA).

---

*Section 5307 of 49 U.S.C.* refers to block grants to finance capital projects and the planning, improvement, and operating costs of equipment, facilities, and associated capital maintenance items for use in mass transportation.

*Section 5309* refers to discretionary grants and loans for capital projects, new and existing fixed guideway systems, an efficient mass transportation system coordinated with other transportation systems, introduction of new technologies, enhancement of urban economic development or incorporation of private investment, and mass transportation projects to meet the needs of the elderly and persons with disabilities.

*Section 5311* refers to financial assistance for non-urbanized areas.

*Section 103(e)(4) of 23 U.S.C.* refers to grants to bus transit systems that operate on Federal-aid highway systems.

---

## 1.1 Regulatory Background

FTA issued its first drug and alcohol testing regulations on February 15, 1994 as two separate rules: 49 CFR Part 653, *Prevention of Prohibited Drug Use in Transit Operations*, and 49 CFR Part 654, *Prevention of Alcohol Misuse in Transit Operations*. The FTA rules were issued in response to *The Omnibus Transportation Employee Testing Act*, enacted by Congress in 1991. They expanded the minimum uniform U.S Department of Transportation (DOT) testing program requirements published earlier in 1994 in 49 CFR Part 40, *Procedures for Transportation Workplace Drug and Alcohol Testing Programs.*

The Omnibus Testing Act was intended to promote the health and safety of transportation employees and the traveling public. It required all DOT administrations to issue regulations requiring funding recipients to perform four types of testing of all safety-sensitive employees for five controlled substances and alcohol, and to establish a prescribed program of rehabilitation and follow-up testing for employees who are given the opportunity to return to safety-sensitive duty after testing positive or refusing to be tested. The Act also required recipients to follow the testing procedures established by the Department of Health and Human Services (DHHS).

DOT revised and reissued Part 40 in 2000, and amended certain provisions in 2003 and 2004. In 2001, FTA issued CFR Part 655, *Prevention of Alcohol Misuse and Prohibited Drug Use in Transit Operations*, to expand the revised department-wide minimum requirements to transit operations. Part 655 supersedes and combines Parts 653 and 654. Per the addition of Section 25 to Part 40 in 2003, a testing event includes test refusals but not canceled tests. The current Part 40 and 655 testing requirements are summarized in Chapter 2 of this report.

## 1.2 Reporting and Certification Requirements

Part 655.72 eliminated the requirement that all direct funding recipients report their drug and alcohol testing program data to FTA annually. It requires that recipients report their data only if requested by FTA. In 2001, FTA developed a stratified random sampling technique to produce an accurate representation of the overall transit industry, in lieu of universal reporting. The intent was to reduce the paperwork burden on a portion of the industry.

Recipients requested to report must do so by March 15. The procedures for reporting in 2003 and the form to be used changed, per the addition of Section 26 and Appendix H of Part 40 (in July 2003). Recipients must either enter the data via internet on the FTA Office of Safety and Security web site: http://transit-safety.volpe.dot.gov/damis. The form, which appears in Appendix C, eliminates some of the previous requirements, but now requires submittal of refusal data by type of refusal for all test types.

All direct recipients must annually prepare and maintain a summary of the results of the DOT-regulated programs that they oversaw during the previous calendar year. All direct recipients must also annually certify regulatory compliance of those programs, and submit the certifications to their FTA regional office.

All grantees must ensure the accuracy and timeliness of each report submitted by their subrecipients. All direct recipients must ensure the accuracy and timeliness of each report submitted by a safety-sensitive contractor or subcontractor.

Failure of a recipient to establish a drug and alcohol testing program and to annually certify regulatory compliance and report information as requested, either in its own operations or in those of a subrecipient or an entity operating on its behalf, may result in the suspension of FTA funding to the recipient. Falsifying compliance information or certifications is a criminal offense.

## 1.3 Reporting Assistance

Assistance on accessing the FTA Office of Safety and Security web site and using the internet reporting system is available from the FTA DAMIS Project Office at (617) 494-6336, FTA.damis@volpe.dot.gov. The FTA Safety and Security Clearinghouse can be reached at (617) 494-2108 for additional copies of this report, as well as previously published annual reports. Other technical assistance materials, including the *Implementation Guidelines for Drug and Alcohol Regulations in Mass Transit* and *Best Practices Manual: FTA Drug and Alcohol Testing Program,* can be obtained from the FTA Safety and Security Clearinghouse, (617) 494-2108, and on the web site: http://transit-safety.volpe.dot.gov/damis.

## 1.4 Data Analysis and Validation

Data submitted for entry in DAMIS are subjected to extensive analysis and validation, both manual and automated. The process entails detailed review of the consistency and reasonableness of the data in each report, identification of errors or questionable entries, and resolution of any problems in consultation with the reporting agencies. This process enables detection and correction of errors of significant magnitude. However, some statistically minor errors may remain.

## 1.5 Organization of Report

The remainder of this report contains five chapters and three appendices:

- *Chapter 2* presents an overview of the current Part 40 and 655 testing requirements, including descriptions of safety-sensitive functions, the types of tests to be performed, and the substances to be tested for.

- *Chapter 3* presents official random drug and alcohol rates for 2003, and compares them with those for 1996 through 2002.

- *Chapter 4* compares the results of the required drug and alcohol tests listed in Chapter 2 and pre-employment alcohol tests. The results are further compared by employer type (transit agencies and contractors), employer size (large, small, and rural), the employee categories listed in Chapter 2, FTA region, and drug type.

- *Chapter 5* summarizes the results of the tests (described in Chapter 2) that are required for employees returned to safety-sensitive duty following a positive test or refusal, using the same categories of comparison as in Chapter 4.

- *Appendix A* lists the terms, and their definitions, associated with the FTA drug and alcohol testing program.

- *Appendix B* lists the ten FTA regions and states they cover.

- *Appendix C* is the MIS data collection form.

# 2. Overview of Part 40 and Part 655 Testing Requirements

This chapter summarizes the requirements of the FTA Drug and Alcohol Testing Program (in Section 2.1) and describes in detail FTA safety-sensitive functions, the tests required by FTA, and the drugs that safety-sensitive employees must be tested for (in Sections 2.2, 2.3, and 2.4, respectively).

## 2.1 Overview of Required Testing Program

Employees who perform any of five safety-sensitive functions must be tested for five controlled substances in four circumstances. Such employees must also be tested for alcohol use in each of those circumstances except pre-employment, though employers may, and many do, require pre-employment tests per Part 40 testing procedures. An additional circumstance (return to duty/follow-up) is required for safety-sensitive employees who are given an opportunity to resume safety-sensitive duties after testing positive for drugs or alcohol or refusing to submit to a required test.

| Safety-Sensitive Employee Categories | Test Types | Drug Types |
|---|---|---|
| Revenue Vehicle Operation | Random | Marijuana |
| Revenue Vehicle and Equipment Maintenance | Post-accident | Cocaine |
| Revenue Vehicle Control/Dispatching | Reasonable suspicion | Phencyclidine (PCP) |
| CDL/Non-Revenue Vehicle | Pre-employment | Opiates |
| Armed Security Personnel | *Return to duty/follow-up | Amphetamines |
| See Section 2.2 for a detailed description of FTA safety-sensitive duties. | See Section 2.3 for a detailed description of tests required by FTA. | See Section 2.4 for a detailed description of the drugs to test for. |

*Required only for employees who test positive for drugs or alcohol or refuse to take a test

Any employee who has a verified positive drug test, has a confirmed alcohol test result of 0.04 or greater, or refuses to submit to a test must be immediately removed from safety-sensitive duty. The employee must then be informed of the resources available for evaluating and resolving problems associated with prohibited drug use and alcohol misuse, including the names, addresses, and telephone numbers of substance abuse professionals (SAPs). The employer then decides which disciplinary action to take. To return the employee to a safety-sensitive function, the employer must ensure that the employee successfully completes a course of treatment prescribed by a SAP and produces a negative return to duty test for drugs or alcohol or both, depending on the evaluation and recommendation of the SAP. Once returned to duty, the employee must continue a treatment program administered by the SAP, which includes a series of follow-up tests.

Part 40, Section 26 and Appendix H (added in 2003) identify four types of drug test refusals and two types of alcohol test refusals:

*Drug test refusal types:*

- Adulterated – submittal of an adulterated specimen
- Substituted – submittal of urine not produced at the collection site
- Shy bladder with no medical explanation – failure to provide enough urine at the collection site, and no medical reason for the failure is found by the medical review officer (MRO)
- Other refusals to submit to testing – Examples include failure to report to the collection site as directed by the employer, leaving the collection site without permission.

*Alcohol test refusal types:*

- Shy lung with no medical explanation – failure to provide enough breath at the collection site, and no medical reason for the failure is found by the MRO
- Other refusals to submit to testing – same examples as for drug tests

Additionally, an employee with a confirmed alcohol concentration of at least 0.02 but less than 0.04 must be removed from duty for at least 8 hours or until a re-test conducted by the employer shows an alcohol concentration of less than 0.02. If the employee is removed from duty for 8 hours, a re-test need not be administered unless the employee exhibits signs of alcohol use upon returning to duty.

Part 40 also prohibits use, manufacture, distribution, dispensing, and possession of all controlled substances by safety-sensitive employees. Furthermore, Parts 40 and 655 prohibit safety-sensitive employees from consuming alcohol in three circumstances:

- While performing a safety-sensitive function
- Four hours before performing a safety-sensitive function unless the employee produces a breath specimen with a concentration below 0.02 (Employees must be given the opportunity to acknowledge use of alcohol in the past 4 hours and to be tested when they arrive for duty.)
- Eight hours following an accident that meets FTA post-accident testing criteria (described in Section 2.3) or until an alcohol test is performed unless the employee's involvement can be completely discounted as a contributing factor to the accident and there were no fatalities

## 2.2 Safety-Sensitive Functions

The **revenue vehicle operation** safety-sensitive job category includes employees who operate a revenue service vehicle, regardless of whether it is in service.

The **revenue vehicle and equipment maintenance** category includes employees who maintain revenue service vehicles or equipment. It also includes many maintenance contract employees who perform routine, ongoing repair or maintenance for FTA recipients and subrecipients that have employees, including supervisors, who perform or could be called upon to perform any of the FTA safety-sensitive functions. Maintenance contractors of 5311 funding recipients are not subject to the testing regulations. Additionally, recipients that operate in areas with a population of 200,000 or less and contract out maintenance services are no longer required to comply.

**Revenue vehicle control/dispatching** includes employees who control the movement of revenue service vehicles. The key consideration is the type of work performed rather than a particular job title. FTA decided not to attempt a universal definition of "dispatchers" in Part 655. Instead, each employer determines whether its particular dispatcher performs or may perform a safety-sensitive function.

**CDL/non-revenue vehicle** includes employees not included in another safety-sensitive category who operate a non-revenue service vehicle (e.g., ancillary vehicle) that requires a Commercial Drivers License (CDL).

**Armed security personnel** are employees who provide security and carry a firearm.

## 2.3 Types of Tests

**Random testing** is considered by FTA to be the most effective deterrent to drug use and alcohol misuse, as well as the most reliable indicator of drug use and alcohol misuse within an employer and in the industry as a whole, provided it is unannounced and unpredictable. Selections for testing must be based on a scientifically valid random-number selection method, to ensure that all safety-sensitive employees have an equal chance of being selected for testing each time a selection is made.

In 2003, the number of random drug tests conducted had to equal a minimum of 50 percent of the average number of safety-sensitive employees in the selection pool, and the number of alcohol tests had to equal a minimum of 10 percent of the pool. These percentages can be amended (per Part 655.45) by the FTA Administrator based on the combined percentage of positive tests plus test refusals, i.e.:

*(verified drug positives + refusals) ÷ (total number of testing events[1])*

*(confirmed alcohol positives[2] + refusals) ÷ (total number of testing events)*

---

[1] Per the addition of Section 26 and Appendix H to Part 40 in 2003, a testing event includes test refusals but not canceled tests.

The testing rate for employers who belong to a consortium applies to the average number of safety-sensitive employees in the consortium's pool. As a result, some individual employers may not appear to meet the random testing requirement, but actually do meet the requirement as long as the consortium, as a whole, tests the minimum number required.

**Post-accident testing** refers to tests required following an accident involving a fatality or an accident that meets any of three other criteria and the employee's involvement cannot be completely discounted as a contributing factor: (1) when a person suffers a bodily injury and immediately receives medical attention away from the scene, (2) when any vehicle involved in the accident incurs damage requiring it to be transported away from the scene by a tow truck or other vehicle, or (3) the mass transit vehicle involved is a rail car, trolley car, trolley bus, or vessel and is removed from revenue service due to the accident.

Employees to be tested include the vehicle operator and any other safety-sensitive employee not in the vehicle whose performance could have contributed to the accident. Both drug and alcohol tests must be administered as soon as possible, but no later than 8 hours after the accident for alcohol and 32 hours for drugs.

**Reasonable suspicion testing** refers to a drug and/or alcohol test that is ordered by a trained supervisor based on specific, contemporaneous, articulable observations concerning the appearance, behavior, speech, or body odor of a safety-sensitive employee.

**Pre-employment testing** refers to testing of candidates for a safety-sensitive position (including existing non-safety-sensitive employees as well as applicants for employment) and for employees who have not performed a safety-sensitive function for more than 90 consecutive calendar days, regardless of the reason, and were removed from the employer's random selection pool during that time. A negative pre-employment test for drugs is required by FTA as a condition for performing safety-sensitive duties under these circumstances. Pre-employment alcohol tests are not required but are permitted under Part 655 providing they are performed in accordance with the testing procedures in Part 40. The alcohol tests are included in the data presented in Chapter 3 because they are conducted per DOT standards and are required by many employers.

The Omnibus Testing Act required a negative pre-employment alcohol test, but FTA suspended the requirement on May 10, 1995, as the result of a U.S. Court of Appeals decision. FTA decided to allow but not require pre-employment alcohol testing in Part 655.

---

[2] A positive alcohol test is a confirmed specimen with a breath alcohol level of at least 0.04.

Part 655 also eliminated the term "hire" in the pre-employment provision. Previously, employers were required to administer a drug test and receive a negative result before hiring an employee. FTA deleted the term to provide employers discretion to administer a pre-employment drug test anytime before an employee first performs a safety-sensitive function and before an employee returns to safety-sensitive duty after being removed from the random pool for an extended period. Part 655 also established a limit, 90 consecutive calendar days, on the amount of time an employee can be removed from the pool without a negative drug test before returning to work.

**Return to duty testing** refers to a drug and/or alcohol test that is required for a safety-sensitive employee who completes a course of treatment prescribed by a SAP after testing positive for drugs or alcohol or refusing to submit to a required test. A negative result for the type (drug or alcohol) of positive or refused test is required before the employee can be returned to duty. SAPs often require the employee to submit to both a drug and an alcohol test even if only one of the tests was at issue.

**Follow-up testing** refers to a drug or alcohol test that is required for an employee who is returned to safety-sensitive duty. The employee is subject to at least six unannounced tests for at least 12 months after returning to duty. The exact number and frequency of tests is prescribed by the SAP, who may order tests for up to 60 months after return to duty. SAPs often require the employee to submit to both a drug and an alcohol test even if only one of the tests was at issue. Follow-up testing is separate from, and in addition to, random testing. Part 655 incorporates follow-up testing under return to duty testing (i.e., return to duty/follow-up testing) as one of five required FTA tests. It was previously listed separately as one of six required FTA tests.

## 2.4  Types of Drugs

**Marijuana** is derived from the hemp plant and comes in a variety of colors such as green, brown, and a gray mixture of leaves. THC or (delta-9-tetrahydrocannabinol) is the primary active chemical in marijuana. It is absorbed quickly into fatty tissues and stored for a long time. The potency and strength of the chemical causes people to use the drug for the mildly tranquilizing, mood and perception-altering effects it produces. The test for marijuana also includes its metabolites.

**Cocaine** is an addictive substance that comes from coca leaves, or is made synthetically. It appears as a white powder that is snorted, ingested, injected, freebased (smoked), or applied directly to the nasal membrane or gums. Cocaine acts as a stimulant to the central nervous system. It gives the user a feeling of exhilaration. The chemicals in cocaine trick the brain into feeling it has experienced pleasure, when in fact it has not.

**Phencyclidine (PCP)**, originally developed as an anesthetic, has adverse side effects that limit its medical use to a tranquilizer for large animals. In people, PCP acts as both a depressant and a hallucinogen, and sometimes as a stimulant. PCP can cause distorted bodily perceptions and a feeling of disassociation where the mind feels separated from the body. These effects can be very upsetting to some people, who may panic as a result.

**Opiates**, also known as narcotic analgesics, include heroin, morphine, and codeine. They are derived from a sap taken from a seedpod of the plant, "papaver somniferum" (or poppy plant). General effects include sedation, slowed reflexes, raspy speech, sluggish movements, slowed breathing, cold skin, and vomiting. The synthetic form of opiates, known as a designer drug, is even more deadly and addictive.

**Amphetamines** include racemic, amphetamine, extroamphetamine, and methamphetamine. They are potent stimulants that can be swallowed, snorted, or injected. They reduce the desire to sleep or eat and can induce a sense of aroused euphoria, accompanied by feelings of increased power, strength, energy, self-assertion, focus, and motivation. Because the body does not readily break down amphetamines, these feelings, which are often intense and ephemeral, may last several hours. Severe mental depression and fatigue can set in when the euphoric feelings wear off.

# 3. Random Drug and Alcohol Rates

As mentioned in Section 2.3, the results of random tests provide the best indication of the overall level of drug use and alcohol misuse, and the combined percentage of positive random tests plus random test refusals are used by FTA in determining minimum random testing rates for the following year. The test result rates for drugs and alcohol, respectively, that are used in determining the random testing rates for the following year are calculated as follows:

*(verified drug positives + refusals) ÷ (total number of testing events[3])*

*(confirmed alcohol positives[4] + refusals) ÷ (total number of testing events)*

## 3.1 Official Random Rates for 2003

The graph at right shows the "official" rates for random drug and random alcohol tests used by the FTA Administrator in determining the random testing rates for 2004. The accompanying table provides the statistical basis for the rates. These data are subdivided by employer type and size, employee category, and FTA region and are compared with data from post-accident, reasonable suspicion, and pre-employment tests in Chapter 4. The refusal data are also subdivided by the types of refusals (defined in Section 2.1) in Chapter 4.

**2003 Random Rates**

DRUGS   ALCOHOL

| | DRUGS | ALCOHOL |
|---|---|---|
| 0.8 | 0.96 | |
| 0.6 | | |
| 0.4 | | |
| 0.2 | | |
| % | | 0.11 |

**Random Tests, Positives, and Refusals**

| | Drugs | Alcohol |
|---|---|---|
| Testing Events | 135,297 | 42,317 |
| Refusals + Positives | 1,299 | 48 |
| Positives | 1,170 | 37 |
| Total Refusals | 129 | 11 |
| Refusal to take test | 83 | 8 |
| Shy Bladder/ Lung | 27 | 3 |
| Adulterated | 15 | N. A. |
| Substituted | 4 | N. A. |
| Refusal Rate | 0.095 | 0.026 |

Because the official random drug rate for 2002 was above 1.0 percent (as shown in the graph in Section 3.2), the random testing rate for drugs remained at 50 percent in 2004, despite the drop below 1.0 percent in 2003. If the rate remains below 1.0 percent in 2004, the FTA Administrator will have the option to reduce the random drug test rate for 2005 to 25 percent of all safety-sensitive employers. Because the 2003 alcohol rate remained well below 0.50 percent, the random testing quota for alcohol remained at 10 percent in 2004.

---

[3] Per the addition of Section 26 to Part 40 in 2003, a testing event includes test refusals but not canceled tests.

[4] A positive alcohol test is a confirmed specimen with a breath alcohol level of at least 0.04.

## 3.2 Official Random Rate Trends

Because the data reporting requirement changed in 2001, the only rates that can be reliably compared for each year of reporting (from 1996 to 2003) are random rates. The results actually reported in 2001 and 2002 did not accurately reflect total FTA testing due to the high proportion of results reported by large employers. The results from random testing were weighted to obtain "official" random rates that reasonably estimate the rate for all persons tested, enabling reliable comparison with the years before 2001 when all employers were required to report. Weighted rates are not available for any test types other than random or any subsets of the random testing.

As shown in the following graph, the official random drug rate dropped in 2003 to the lowest rate (0.96 percent) since employers in all size categories were required to report, following its only rise (in 2002). The 2003 rate was 40 percent lower than the rate in 1996.

As also shown in the next graph, the official random alcohol rate dropped by 50 percent in 2003 to 0.11 percent, by far the lowest rate since employers in all size categories were required to report.

**Official Random Drug and Alcohol Test Rates: 1996 to 2003**

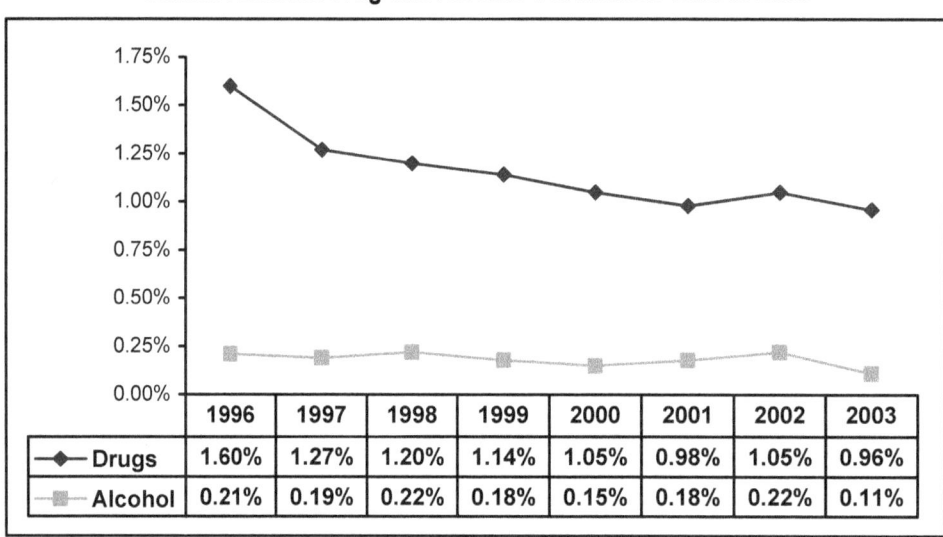

|  | 1996 | 1997 | 1998 | 1999 | 2000 | 2001 | 2002 | 2003 |
|---|---|---|---|---|---|---|---|---|
| Drugs | 1.60% | 1.27% | 1.20% | 1.14% | 1.05% | 0.98% | 1.05% | 0.96% |
| Alcohol | 0.21% | 0.19% | 0.22% | 0.18% | 0.15% | 0.18% | 0.22% | 0.11% |

# 4. Drug and Alcohol Data for Four Required Test Types

This chapter presents data from the four circumstances cited in Chapter 2 that must be performed by all employers subject to Part 655[5]: random, post-accident, reasonable suspicion, and pre-employment. Data from the other testing circumstance cited in Chapter 2 (return to duty tests and follow-up tests) are presented separately (in Chapter 5) from data for the other four test types because that test type represents a different segment of the test population—specimens produced by persons who have already been removed from duty for drug or alcohol violations and have completed a rehabilitation program—and not all employers offer rehabilitation.

The following two charts compare the combined percentage of positive tests plus test refusals and the percentages of total drug tests reported in 2003 for each of the four test types. The two charts on the next page compare the combined percentage of positive tests plus test refusals and percentages of total alcohol tests reported in 2003 for each of the four test types. The combined percentages of positive tests plus refusals are calculated as follows:

*(verified drug positives + refusals) ÷ (total number of testing events[6])*

*(confirmed alcohol positives[7] + refusals) ÷ (total number of testing events)*

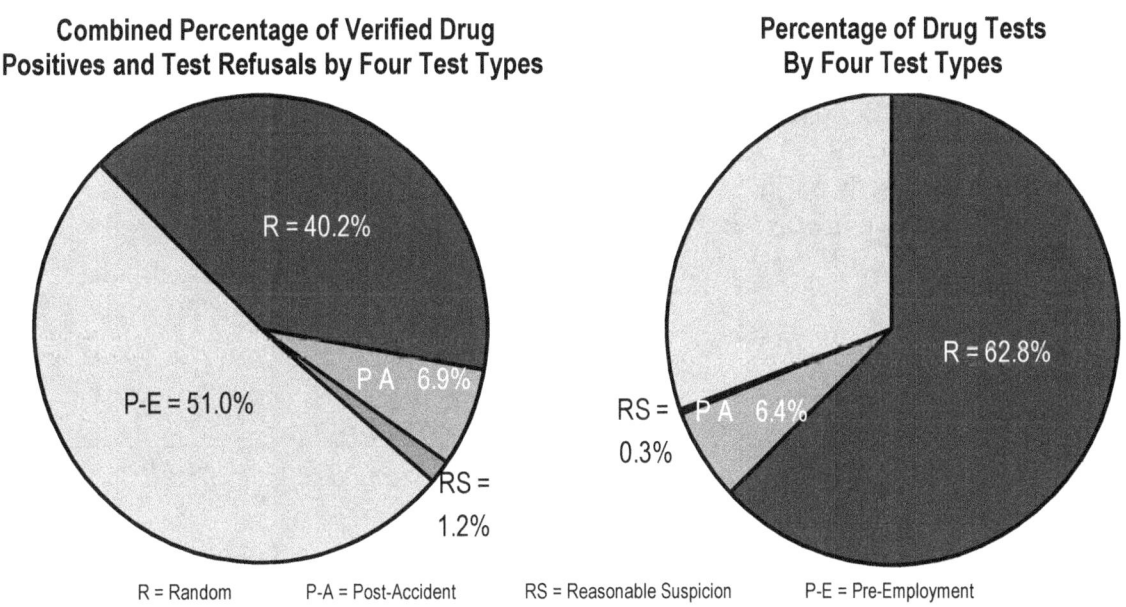

| **Combined Percentage of Verified Drug Positives and Test Refusals by Four Test Types** | **Percentage of Drug Tests By Four Test Types** |

R = Random    P-A = Post-Accident    RS = Reasonable Suspicion    P-E = Pre-Employment

---

[5] Part 655 does not require pre-employment alcohol testing. It is included in this chapter because many employers require it, and Part 655 requires that the data be reported if the tests are performed.

[6] Per the addition of Section 26 and Appendix H to Part 40 in 2003, a testing event includes test refusals but not canceled tests.

[7] A positive alcohol test is a confirmation test with a breath alcohol level of at least 0.04.

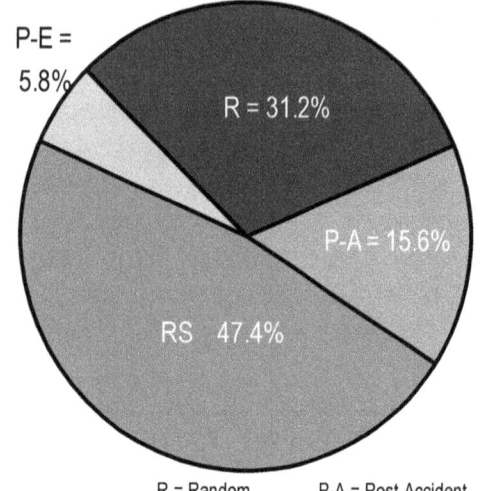

**Combined Percentage of Confirmed Alcohol Positives and Test Refusals by Four Test Types**

P-E = 5.8%

R = 31.2%

P-A = 15.6%

RS  47.4%

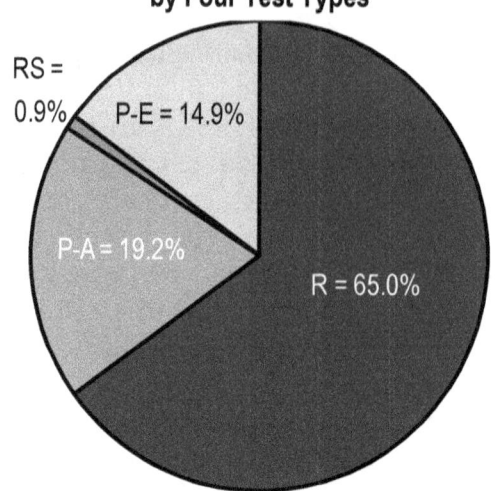

**Percentage of Alcohol Tests by Four Test Types**

RS = 0.9%

P-E = 14.9%

P-A = 19.2%

R = 65.0%

R = Random    P-A = Post-Accident    RS = Reasonable Suspicion    P-E = Pre-Employment

The rates[8] for each of the four test types and for the four types combined, for both drugs and alcohol, appear in the graph at right. The table below provides the statistical basis for the rates. These data are subdivided by employer type and size, employee category, FTA region, and type of drug in Sections 4.1, 4.2, 4.3, and 4.4, respectively. Confirmed alcohol specimens between 0.02 and 0.039 are presented by test type in Section 4.5 and are subdivided by employer type, employer size, employee category, and FTA region.

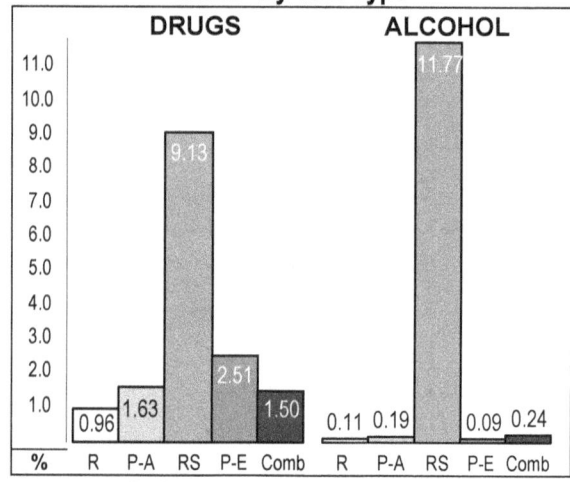

**Rates[8] by Test Type**

R = Random    P-A = Post-Accident
RS = Reasonable Suspicion    P-E = Pre-Employment    Comb = Combined

### Tests, Positives, and Refusals by Test Type

| | Drugs | | | | | Alcohol | | | | |
|---|---|---|---|---|---|---|---|---|---|---|
| | Random | Post-Accident | Reasonable Suspicion | Pre-Employment | Total | Random | Post-Accident | Reasonable Suspicion | Pre-Employment | Total |
| Testing Events | 135,297 | 13,715 | 657 | 65,774 | 215,443 | 42,317 | 12,490 | 620 | 9,672 | 65,099 |
| Refusals + Positives | 1,299 | 224 | 60 | 1,651 | 3,234 | 48 | 24 | 73 | 9 | 154 |
| Positives | 1,170 | 204 | 55 | 1,562 | 2,991 | 37 | 10 | 68 | 8 | 123 |
| Total Refusals | 129 | 20 | 5 | 89 | 243 | 11 | 14 | 5 | 1 | 31 |
| Refusal to take test | 83 | 16 | 4 | 59 | 162 | 8 | 11 | 5 | 0 | 24 |
| Shy Bladder/Lung | 27 | 2 | 1 | 4 | 34 | 3 | 3 | 0 | 1 | 7 |
| Adulterated | 15 | 0 | 0 | 15 | 30 | N. A. | N. A. | N. A. | N. A. | N. A. |
| Substituted | 4 | 2 | 0 | 11 | 17 | N. A. | N. A. | N. A. | N. A. | N. A. |
| Refusal Rate | 0.095 | 0.146 | 0.761 | 0.135 | 0.113 | 0.026 | 0.112 | 0.806 | 0.010 | 0.048 |

---

[8] The rates in all of the graphs are the combined percentages of positive tests plus test refusals.

## 4.1 Data for Four Test Types by Employer Type and Size

The data above are subdivided by employer type, by employer size, and by employer size and type combined, respectively, in this section. The rates for each data set are shown in a separate pair of graphs. Each graph pair is followed by a table or tables that provide the statistical basis for the rates.

Because all of the alcohol rates by employer type except reasonable suspicion are less than 0.5 percent, the space below "0.5" in the following alcohol graph is expanded under the divider line to allow greater clarity.

**Rates by Test Type and Employer Type**

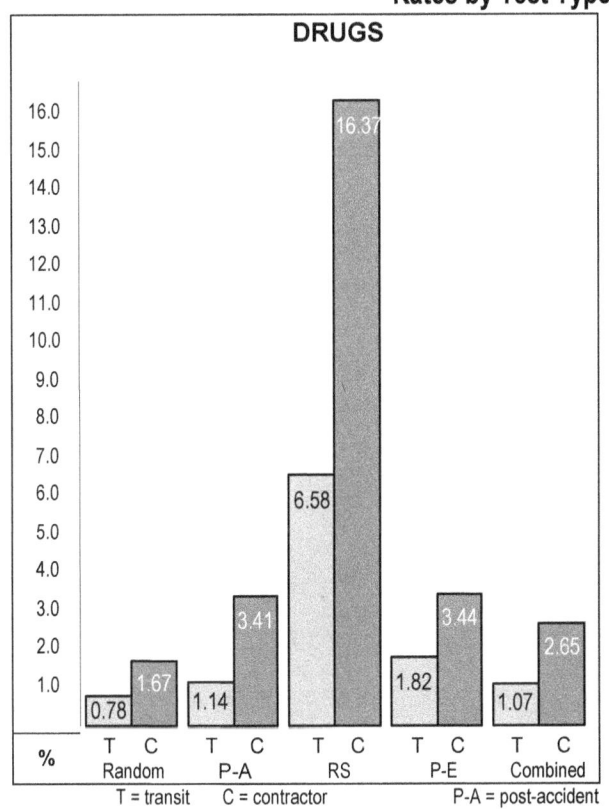

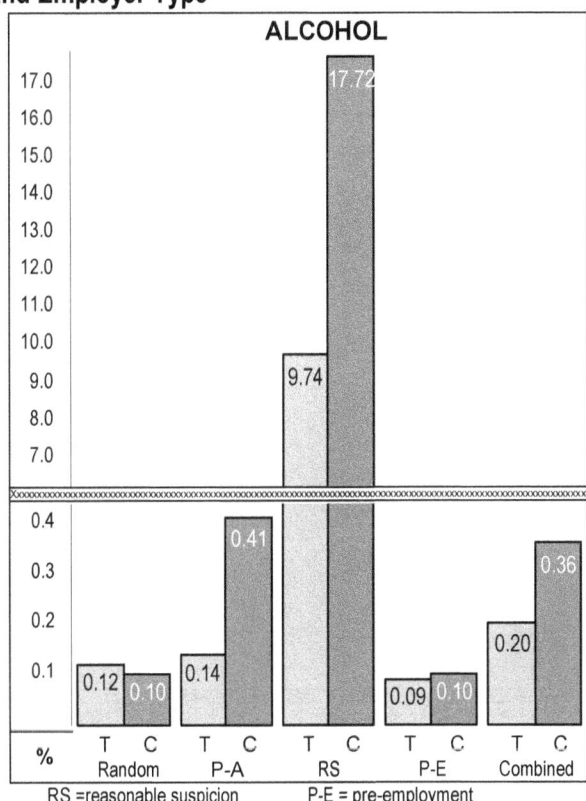

### Tests, Positives, and Refusals by Test Type and Employer Type

| | Drugs | | | | | | | | | |
|---|---|---|---|---|---|---|---|---|---|---|
| | Random | | Post-Accident | | Reasonable Suspicion | | Pre-Employment | | Total | |
| | Transit | Contractor | Transit | Contractor | Transit | Contractor | Transit | Contractor | Transit | Contractor |
| Testing Events | 108,239 | 27,058 | 10,753 | 2,962 | 486 | 171 | 37,597 | 28,177 | 157,075 | 58,368 |
| Refusals + Positives | 847 | 452 | 123 | 101 | 32 | 28 | 683 | 968 | 1,685 | 1,549 |
| Positives | 771 | 399 | 115 | 89 | 28 | 27 | 655 | 907 | 1,569 | 1,422 |
| Total Refusals | 76 | 53 | 8 | 12 | 4 | 1 | 28 | 61 | 116 | 127 |
| Refusal to take test | 47 | 36 | 5 | 11 | 3 | 1 | 19 | 40 | 74 | 88 |
| Shy Bladder | 19 | 8 | 1 | 1 | 1 | 0 | 1 | 3 | 22 | 12 |
| Adulterated | 6 | 9 | 0 | 0 | 0 | 0 | 4 | 11 | 10 | 20 |
| Substituted | 4 | 0 | 2 | 0 | 0 | 0 | 3 | 8 | 9 | 8 |
| Refusal Rate | 0.070 | 0.196 | 0.074 | 0.405 | 0.823 | 0.585 | 0.074 | 0.216 | 0.074 | 0.218 |

## Tests, Positives, and Refusals by Test Type and Employer Type

| | Alcohol | | | | | | | | | |
|---|---|---|---|---|---|---|---|---|---|---|
| | Random | | Post-Accident | | Reasonable Suspicion | | Pre-Employment | | Total | |
| | Transit | Contractor | Transit | Contractor | Transit | Contractor | Transit | Contractor | Transit | Contractor |
| Testing Events | 34,446 | 7,871 | 10,038 | 2,452 | 462 | 158 | 6,650 | 3,022 | 51,596 | 13,503 |
| Refusals + Positives | 40 | 8 | 14 | 10 | 45 | 28 | 6 | 3 | 105 | 49 |
| Positives | 32 | 5 | 8 | 2 | 44 | 24 | 5 | 3 | 89 | 34 |
| Total Refusals | 8 | 3 | 6 | 8 | 1 | 4 | 1 | 0 | 16 | 15 |
| Refusal to take test | 5 | 3 | 3 | 8 | 1 | 4 | 0 | 0 | 9 | 15 |
| Shy Lung | 3 | 0 | 3 | 0 | 0 | 0 | 1 | 0 | 7 | 0 |
| Refusal Rate | 0.023 | 0.038 | 0.060 | 0.326 | 0.216 | 2.532 | 0.015 | 0 | 0.031 | 0.111 |

Because the reasonable suspicion drug rates by employer size are much higher than those for the other types, separate scales are used in the following graph.

## Rates by Test Type and Employer Size

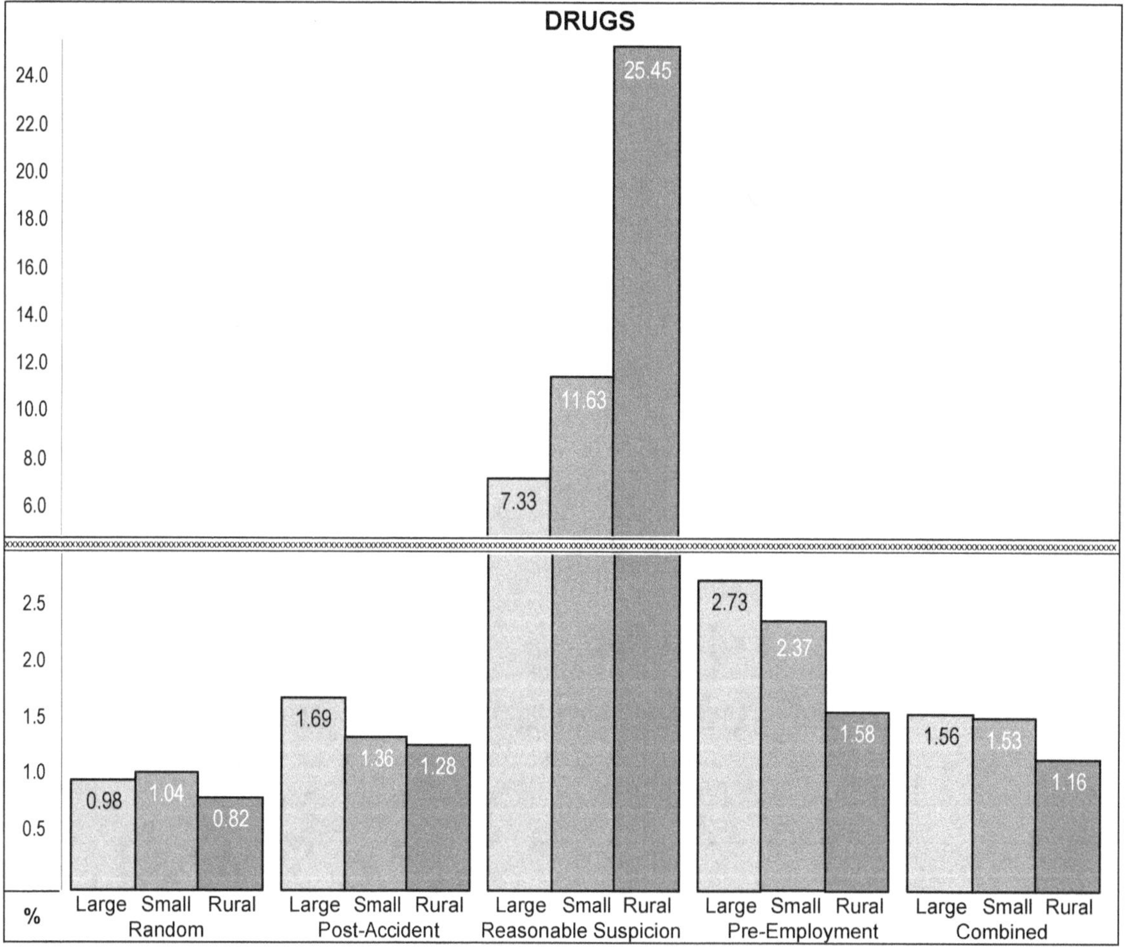

DRUGS

Because all of the alcohol rates by employer size except reasonable suspicion are less than 0.3 percent, the space below "0.3" in the following alcohol graph is expanded under the divider line to allow greater clarity.

## Rates by Test Type and Employer Size

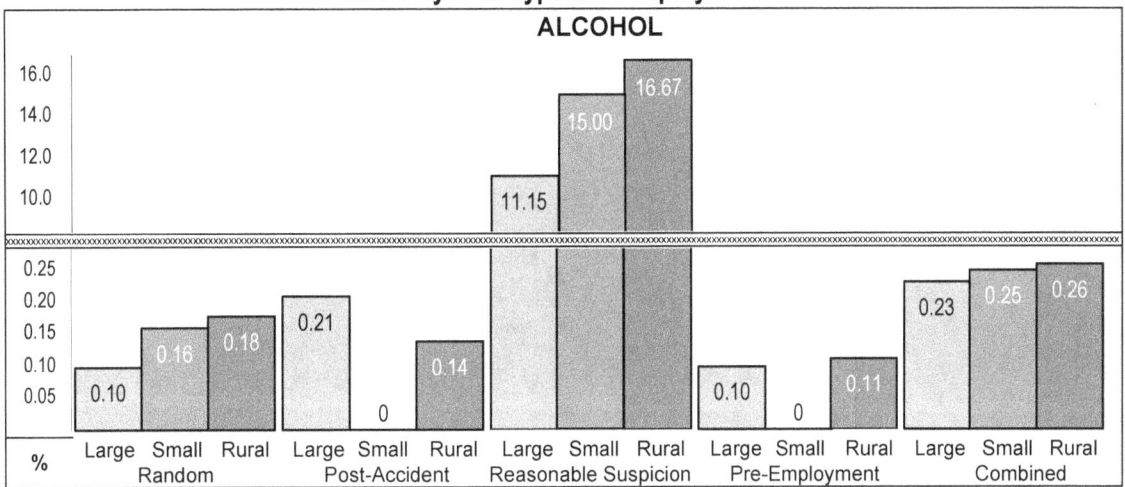

## Tests, Positives, and Refusals by Test Type and Employer Size

| | Drugs | | | | | | | | | | | | | | |
|---|---|---|---|---|---|---|---|---|---|---|---|---|---|---|---|
| | Random | | | Post-Accident | | | Reasonable Suspicion | | | Pre-Employment | | | Total | | |
| | Large | Small | Rural | Large | Small | Rural | Large | Small | Rural | Large | Small | Rural | Large | Small | Rural |
| TE | 108,735 | 8,556 | 18,006 | 11,592 | 1,104 | 1,019 | 559 | 43 | 55 | 49,860 | 4,678 | 11,236 | 170,746 | 14,381 | 30,316 |
| R+P | 1,063 | 89 | 147 | 196 | 15 | 13 | 41 | 5 | 14 | 1,363 | 111 | 177 | 2,663 | 220 | 351 |
| P | 967 | 76 | 127 | 178 | 13 | 13 | 39 | 5 | 11 | 1,290 | 102 | 170 | 2,474 | 196 | 321 |
| TR | 96 | 13 | 20 | 18 | 2 | 0 | 2 | 0 | 3 | 73 | 9 | 7 | 189 | 24 | 30 |
| RTT | 60 | 7 | 16 | 14 | 2 | 0 | 1 | 0 | 3 | 50 | 5 | 4 | 125 | 14 | 23 |
| SB | 18 | 6 | 3 | 2 | 0 | 0 | 1 | 0 | 0 | 2 | 1 | 1 | 23 | 7 | 4 |
| Adul | 14 | 0 | 1 | 0 | 0 | 0 | 0 | 0 | 0 | 15 | 0 | 0 | 29 | 0 | 1 |
| Sub | 4 | 0 | 0 | 2 | 0 | 0 | 0 | 0 | 0 | 6 | 3 | 2 | 12 | 3 | 2 |
| R Rate | 0.088 | 0.152 | 0.111 | 0.155 | 0.181 | 0.000 | 0.358 | 0.000 | 5.455 | 0.146 | 0.192 | 0.062 | 0.111 | 0.167 | 0.099 |

| | Alcohol | | | | | | | | | | | | | | |
|---|---|---|---|---|---|---|---|---|---|---|---|---|---|---|---|
| | Random | | | Post-Accident | | | Reasonable Suspicion | | | Pre-Employment | | | Total | | |
| | Large | Small | Rural | Large | Small | Rural | Large | Small | Rural | Large | Small | Rural | Large | Small | Rural |
| TE | 34,699 | 2,530 | 5,088 | 10,853 | 899 | 738 | 538 | 40 | 42 | 8,290 | 456 | 926 | 54,380 | 3,925 | 6,794 |
| R+P | 35 | 4 | 9 | 23 | 0 | 1 | 60 | 6 | 7 | 8 | 0 | 1 | 126 | 10 | 18 |
| P | 29 | 4 | 4 | 10 | 0 | 0 | 56 | 6 | 6 | 7 | 0 | 1 | 102 | 10 | 11 |
| TR | 6 | 0 | 5 | 13 | 0 | 1 | 4 | 0 | 1 | 1 | 0 | 0 | 24 | 0 | 7 |
| RTT | 4 | 0 | 4 | 11 | 0 | 0 | 4 | 0 | 1 | 0 | 0 | 0 | 19 | 0 | 5 |
| SL | 2 | 0 | 1 | 2 | 0 | 1 | 0 | 0 | 0 | 1 | 0 | 0 | 5 | 0 | 2 |
| R Rate | 0.017 | 0.000 | 0.098 | 0.120 | 0.000 | 0.136 | 0.743 | 0.000 | 2.381 | 0.012 | 0 | 0 | 0.044 | 0.000 | 0.103 |

TE = testing events    P = positives    R = refusals    TR = total refusals    R Rate = refusal rate

RTT = refusal to take test    SL = shy lung    SB = shy bladder    Adul = adulterated    Sub = substituted

Because four of the reasonable suspicion drug rates by employer size and employer type are much higher than those for the other types, the reasonable suspicion rates are presented on separate scales in the following graph.

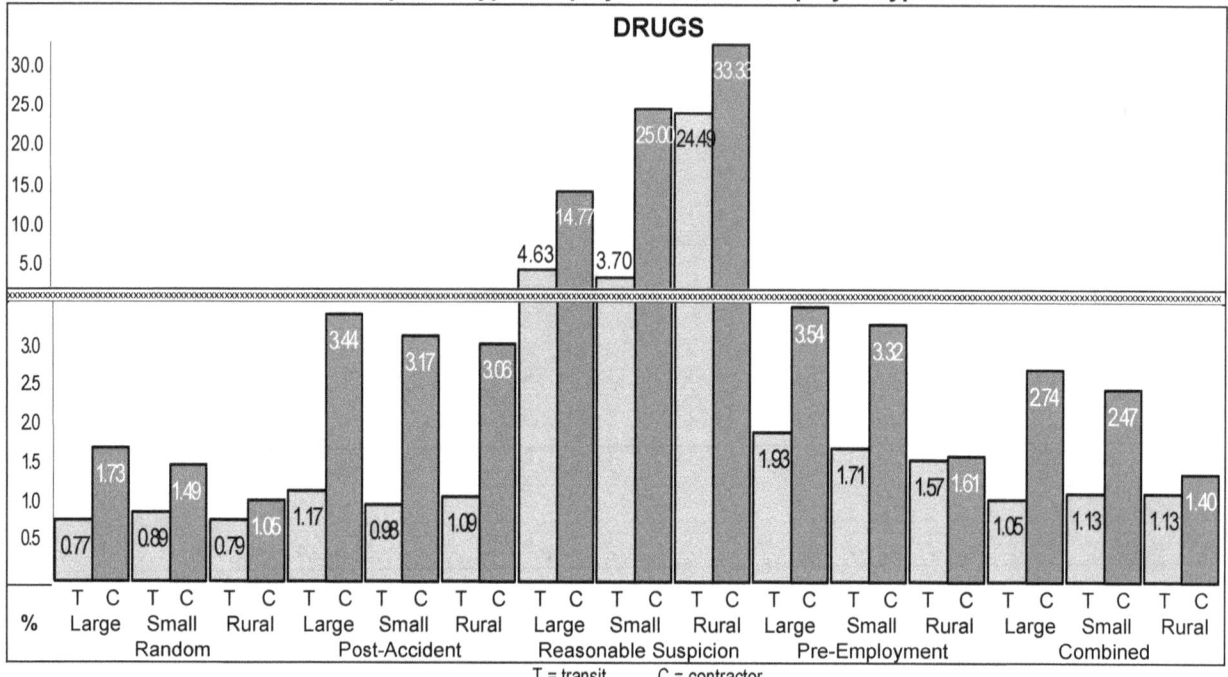

Because all of the alcohol rates by employer size and employer type except the reasonable suspicion rates are less than 0.5 percent, the space below "0.5" in the following alcohol graph is expanded under the divider line to allow greater clarity. Additionally, *the following graph does not contain columns for employer size that show a rate of "0" in the preceding test type/employer size graph.*

Rates by Test Type, Employer Size, and Employer Type

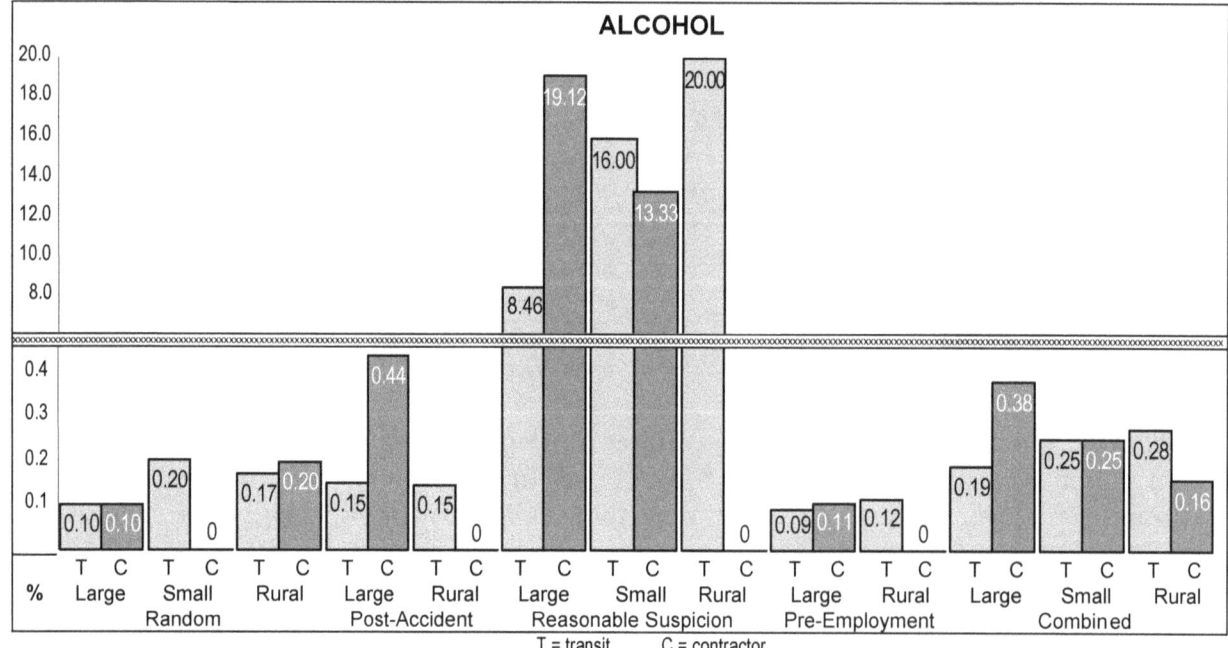

## Tests, Positives, and Refusals by Test Type, Employer Size, and Employer Type

| | | Drugs | | | | | | Alcohol | | | | | |
|---|---|---|---|---|---|---|---|---|---|---|---|---|---|
| | | Large | | Small | | Rural | | Large | | Small | | Rural | |
| | | Transit | Contractor | Transit | Contractor | Transit | Contractor | Transit | Contractor | Transit | Contractor | Transit | Contractor |
| Random | TE | 85,550 | 23,185 | 6,405 | 2,151 | 16,284 | 1,722 | 27,875 | 6,824 | 1,974 | 557 | 4,597 | 491 |
| | R+P | 661 | 402 | 57 | 32 | 129 | 18 | 28 | 7 | 4 | 0 | 8 | 1 |
| | P | 611 | 356 | 51 | 25 | 109 | 18 | 25 | 4 | 4 | 0 | 3 | 1 |
| | TR | 50 | 46 | 6 | 7 | 20 | 0 | 3 | 3 | 0 | 0 | 5 | 0 |
| | RTT | 26 | 34 | 5 | 2 | 16 | 0 | 1 | 3 | 0 | 0 | 4 | 0 |
| | SB | 15 | 3 | 1 | 5 | 3 | 0 | 2 | 0 | 0 | 0 | 1 | 0 |
| | Adul | 5 | 9 | 0 | 0 | 1 | 0 | N. A. | N. A. | N. A. | N. A. | N. A. | N. A. |
| | Sub | 4 | 0 | 0 | 0 | 0 | 0 | N. A. | N. A. | N. A. | N. A. | N. A. | N. A. |
| | R Rate | 0.058 | 0.198 | 0.094 | 0.325 | 0.123 | 0 | 0.011 | 0.044 | 0 | 0 | 0.109 | 0 |
| Post-Accident | TE | 8,917 | 2,675 | 915 | 189 | 921 | 98 | 8,578 | 2,275 | 780 | 119 | 680 | 58 |
| | R+P | 104 | 92 | 9 | 6 | 10 | 3 | 13 | 10 | 0 | 0 | 1 | 0 |
| | P | 96 | 82 | 9 | 4 | 10 | 3 | 8 | 2 | 0 | 0 | 0 | 0 |
| | TR | 8 | 10 | 0 | 2 | 0 | 0 | 5 | 8 | 0 | 0 | 1 | 0 |
| | RTT | 5 | 9 | 0 | 2 | 0 | 0 | 3 | 8 | 0 | 0 | 0 | 0 |
| | SB | 1 | 1 | 0 | 0 | 0 | 0 | 2 | 0 | 0 | 0 | 1 | 0 |
| | Adul | 0 | 0 | 0 | 0 | 0 | 0 | N. A. | N. A. | N. A. | N. A. | N. A. | N. A. |
| | Sub | 2 | 0 | 0 | 0 | 0 | 0 | N. A. | N. A. | N. A. | N. A. | N. A. | N. A. |
| | R Rate | 0.090 | 0.374 | 0 | 1.058 | 0 | 0 | 0.058 | 0.352 | 0 | 0 | 0.147 | 0 |
| Reasonable Suspicion | TE | 410 | 149 | 27 | 16 | 49 | 6 | 402 | 136 | 25 | 15 | 35 | 7 |
| | R+P | 19 | 22 | 1 | 4 | 12 | 2 | 34 | 26 | 4 | 2 | 7 | 0 |
| | P | 18 | 21 | 1 | 4 | 9 | 2 | 34 | 22 | 4 | 2 | 6 | 0 |
| | TR | 1 | 1 | 0 | 0 | 3 | 0 | 0 | 4 | 0 | 0 | 1 | 0 |
| | RTT | 0 | 1 | 0 | 0 | 3 | 0 | 0 | 4 | 0 | 0 | 1 | 0 |
| | SB | 1 | 0 | 0 | 0 | 0 | 0 | 0 | 0 | 0 | 0 | 0 | 0 |
| | Adul | 0 | 0 | 0 | 0 | 0 | 0 | N. A. | N. A. | N. A. | N. A. | N. A. | N. A. |
| | Sub | 0 | 0 | 0 | 0 | 0 | 0 | N. A. | N. A. | N. A. | N. A. | N. A. | N. A. |
| | R Rate | 0.244 | 0.671 | 0 | 0 | 6.122 | 0 | 0 | 2.941 | 0 | 0 | 2.857 | 0 |
| Pre-Employment | TE | 24,855 | 25,005 | 2,750 | 1,928 | 9,992 | 1,244 | 5,439 | 2,851 | 362 | 94 | 849 | 77 |
| | R+P | 479 | 884 | 47 | 64 | 157 | 20 | 5 | 3 | 0 | 0 | 1 | 0 |
| | P | 462 | 828 | 42 | 60 | 151 | 19 | 4 | 3 | 0 | 0 | 1 | 0 |
| | TR | 17 | 56 | 5 | 4 | 6 | 1 | 1 | 0 | 0 | 0 | 0 | 0 |
| | RTT | 12 | 38 | 3 | 2 | 4 | 0 | 0 | 0 | 0 | 0 | 0 | 0 |
| | SB | 0 | 2 | 0 | 1 | 1 | 0 | 1 | 0 | 0 | 0 | 0 | 0 |
| | Adul | 4 | 11 | 0 | 0 | 0 | 0 | N. A. | N. A. | N. A. | N. A. | N. A. | N. A. |
| | Sub | 1 | 5 | 2 | 1 | 1 | 1 | N. A. | N. A. | N. A. | N. A. | N. A. | N. A. |
| | R Rate | 0.068 | 0.224 | 0.182 | 0.207 | 0.060 | 0.080 | 0.018 | 0 | 0 | 0 | 0 | 0 |
| Total | TE | 119,732 | 51,014 | 10,097 | 4,284 | 27,246 | 3,070 | 42,294 | 12,086 | 3,141 | 785 | 6,161 | 633 |
| | R+P | 1,263 | 1,400 | 114 | 106 | 308 | 43 | 80 | 46 | 8 | 2 | 17 | 1 |
| | P | 1,263 | 1,400 | 114 | 106 | 308 | 43 | 80 | 46 | 8 | 2 | 17 | 1 |
| | TR | 1,187 | 1,287 | 103 | 93 | 279 | 42 | 71 | 31 | 8 | 2 | 10 | 1 |
| | RTT | 43 | 82 | 8 | 6 | 23 | 0 | 4 | 15 | 0 | 0 | 5 | 0 |
| | SB | 17 | 6 | 1 | 6 | 4 | 0 | 5 | 0 | 0 | 0 | 2 | 0 |
| | Adul | 9 | 20 | 0 | 0 | 1 | 0 | N. A. | N. A. | N. A. | N. A. | N. A. | N. A. |
| | Sub | 7 | 5 | 2 | 1 | 1 | 1 | N. A. | N. A. | N. A. | N. A. | N. A. | N. A. |
| | R Rate | 0.063 | 0.222 | 0.109 | 0.303 | 0.106 | 0.033 | 0.021 | 0.124 | 0 | 0 | 0.114 | 0.000 |

RVO = Revenue Vehicle Operation  RV&EM = Revenue Vehicle and Equipment Maintenance
RVC/D = Revenue Vehicle Control/Dispatching  CDL/N-RV = CDL/Non-Revenue Vehicle  ASP = Armed Security Personnel
TE = testing events  P = positives  R = refusals  TR = total refusals  R Rate = refusal rate
RTT = refusal to take test  SB = shy bladder  Adul = adulterated  Sub = substituted

## 4.2 Data for Four Test Types by Employee Category

The next two graphs show the rates for each test type, as well as the rates for all four types combined, by employee category for drug tests and for alcohol tests, respectively. Because all of the alcohol rates except reasonable suspicion are less than 0.6 percent, the space below "0.6" in the alcohol graph is expanded under the divider line to allow greater clarity. The table on the next page provides the statistical basis for the rates. These data are subdivided by employer type and by employer size later in this section.

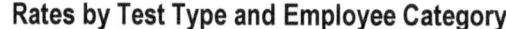

### Rates by Test Type and Employee Category

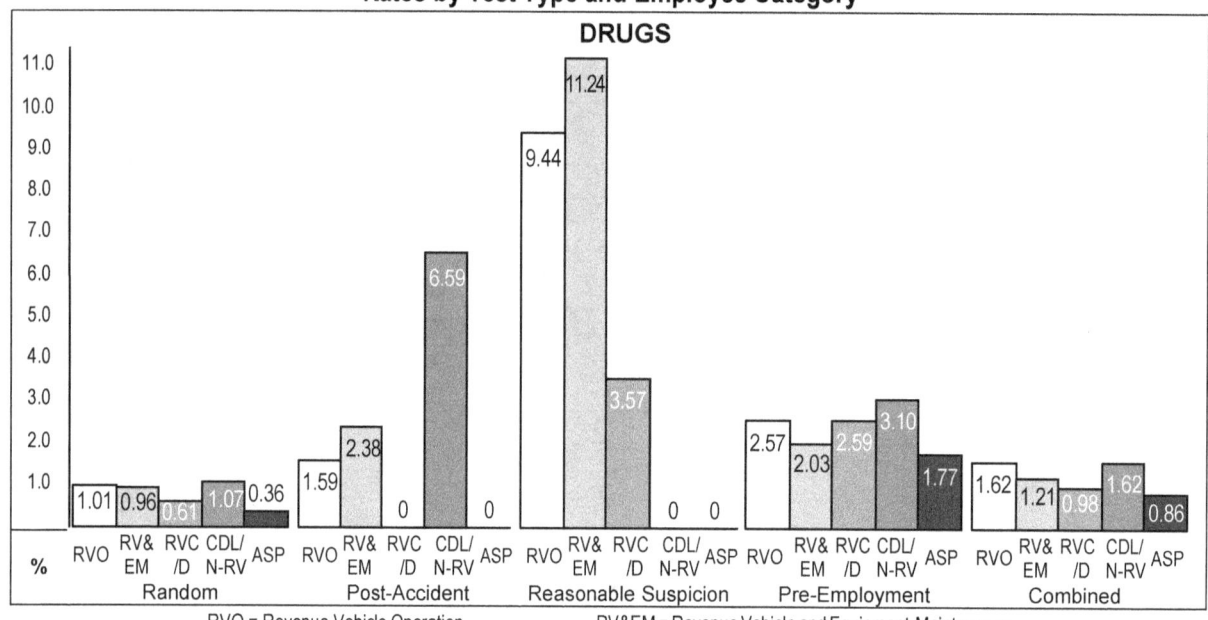

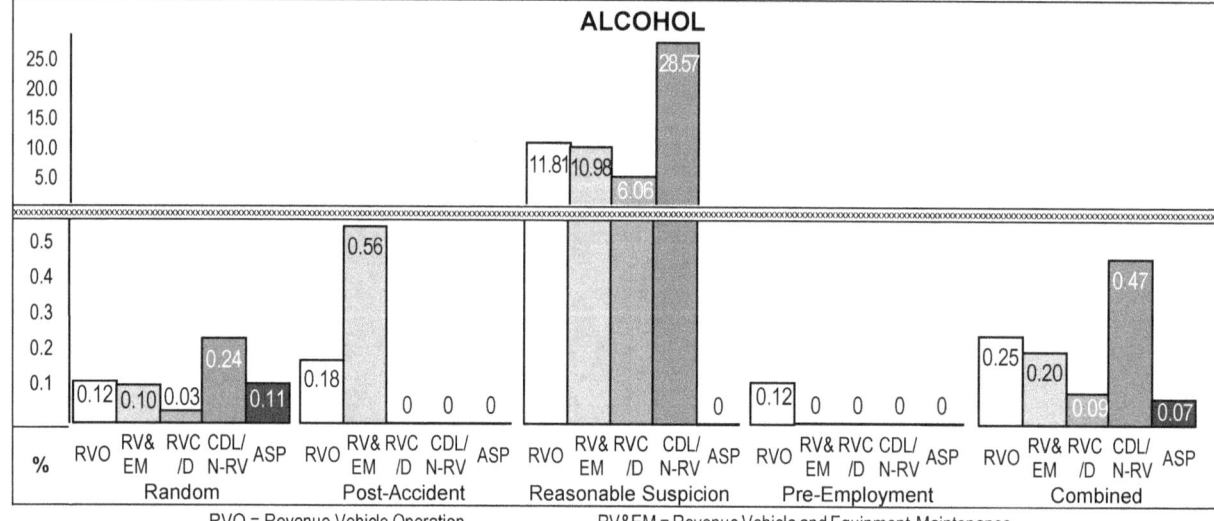

## Tests, Positives, and Refusals by Test Type and Employee Category

| | | Drugs | | | | | Alcohol | | | | |
|---|---|---|---|---|---|---|---|---|---|---|---|
| | | RVO | RV&EM | RVC/D | CDL/N-RV | ASP | RVO | RV&EM | RVC/D | CDL/N-RV | ASP |
| Random | TE | 92,496 | 27,602 | 9,515 | 3,189 | 2,495 | 28,702 | 8,587 | 2,882 | 1,254 | 892 |
| | R+P | 932 | 266 | 58 | 34 | 9 | 34 | 9 | 1 | 3 | 1 |
| | P | 843 | 240 | 50 | 32 | 5 | 24 | 9 | 0 | 3 | 1 |
| | TR | 89 | 26 | 8 | 2 | 4 | 10 | 0 | 1 | 0 | 0 |
| | RTT | 55 | 19 | 5 | 0 | 4 | 7 | 0 | 1 | 0 | 0 |
| | SB | 22 | 2 | 1 | 2 | 0 | 3 | 0 | 0 | 0 | 0 |
| | Adul | 10 | 3 | 2 | 0 | 0 | N. A. | N. A. | N. A. | N. A. | N. A. |
| | Sub | 2 | 2 | 0 | 0 | 0 | N. A. | N. A. | N. A. | N. A. | N. A. |
| | R Rate | 0.096 | 0.094 | 0.084 | 0.063 | 0.160 | 0.035 | 0 | 0.035 | 0 | 0 |
| Post-Accident | TE | 12,783 | 630 | 107 | 91 | 104 | 11,719 | 539 | 89 | 79 | 64 |
| | R+P | 203 | 15 | 0 | 6 | 0 | 21 | 3 | 0 | 0 | 0 |
| | P | 185 | 13 | 0 | 6 | 0 | 10 | 0 | 0 | 0 | 0 |
| | TR | 18 | 2 | 0 | 0 | 0 | 11 | 3 | 0 | 0 | 0 |
| | RTT | 14 | 2 | 0 | 0 | 0 | 9 | 2 | 0 | 0 | 0 |
| | SB | 2 | 0 | 0 | 0 | 0 | 2 | 1 | 0 | 0 | 0 |
| | Adul | 0 | 0 | 0 | 0 | 0 | N. A. | N. A. | N. A. | N. A. | N. A. |
| | Sub | 2 | 0 | 0 | 0 | 0 | N. A. | N. A. | N. A. | N. A. | N. A. |
| | R Rate | 0.141 | 0.317 | 0 | 0 | 0 | 0.094 | 0.557 | 0 | 0 | 0 |
| Reasonable Suspicion | TE | 519 | 89 | 28 | 20 | 1 | 491 | 82 | 33 | 14 | 0 |
| | R+P | 49 | 10 | 1 | 0 | 0 | 58 | 9 | 2 | 4 | 0 |
| | P | 46 | 9 | 0 | 0 | 0 | 56 | 7 | 1 | 4 | 0 |
| | TR | 3 | 1 | 1 | 0 | 0 | 2 | 2 | 1 | 0 | 0 |
| | RTT | 2 | 1 | 1 | 0 | 0 | 2 | 2 | 1 | 0 | 0 |
| | SB | 1 | 0 | 0 | 0 | 0 | 0 | 0 | 0 | 0 | 0 |
| | Adul | 0 | 0 | 0 | 0 | 0 | N. A. | N. A. | N. A. | N. A. | N. A. |
| | Sub | 0 | 0 | 0 | 0 | 0 | N. A. | N. A. | N. A. | N. A. | N. A. |
| | R Rate | 0.578 | 1.124 | 3.571 | 0 | 0 | 0.407 | 2.439 | 3.030 | 0 | 0 |
| Pre-Employment | TE | 54,936 | 6,271 | 2,197 | 903 | 1,467 | 7,671 | 1,120 | 285 | 154 | 442 |
| | R+P | 1,413 | 127 | 57 | 28 | 26 | 9 | 0 | 0 | 0 | 0 |
| | P | 1,339 | 122 | 53 | 24 | 24 | 8 | 0 | 0 | 0 | 0 |
| | TR | 74 | 5 | 4 | 4 | 2 | 1 | 0 | 0 | 0 | 0 |
| | RTT | 47 | 4 | 3 | 3 | 2 | 0 | 0 | 0 | 0 | 0 |
| | SB | 3 | 1 | 0 | 0 | 0 | 1 | 0 | 0 | 0 | 0 |
| | Adul | 13 | 0 | 1 | 1 | 0 | N. A. | N. A | N. A. | N. A. | N. A. |
| | Sub | 11 | 0 | 0 | 0 | 0 | N. A. | N. A. | N. A. | N. A. | N. A. |
| | R Rate | 0.135 | 0.080 | 0.182 | 0.443 | 0.136 | 0.013 | 0 | 0 | 0 | 0 |
| Total | TE | 160,734 | 34,592 | 11,847 | 4,203 | 4,067 | 48,583 | 10,328 | 3,289 | 1,501 | 1,398 |
| | R+P | 2,597 | 418 | 116 | 68 | 35 | 122 | 21 | 3 | 7 | 1 |
| | P | 2,413 | 384 | 103 | 62 | 29 | 98 | 16 | 1 | 7 | 1 |
| | TR | 184 | 34 | 13 | 6 | 6 | 24 | 5 | 2 | 0 | 0 |
| | RTT | 118 | 26 | 9 | 3 | 6 | 18 | 4 | 2 | 0 | 0 |
| | SB | 28 | 3 | 1 | 2 | 0 | 6 | 1 | 0 | 0 | 0 |
| | Adul | 23 | 3 | 3 | 1 | 0 | N. A. | N. A. | N. A. | N. A. | N. A. |
| | Sub | 15 | 2 | 0 | 0 | 0 | N. A. | N. A. | N. A. | N. A. | N. A. |
| | R Rate | 0.114 | 0.098 | 0.110 | 0.143 | 0.148 | 0.049 | 0.048 | 0.061 | 0 | 0 |

RVO = Revenue Vehicle Operation  RV&EM = Revenue Vehicle and Equipment Maintenance
RVC/D = Revenue Vehicle Control/Dispatching  CDL/N-RV = CDL/Non-Revenue Vehicle  ASP = Armed Security Personnel
TE = testing events  P = positives  R = refusals  TR = total refusals  R Rate = refusal rate
RTT = refusal to take test  SB = shy bladder  Adul = adulterated  Sub = substituted

### 4.2.1 Data for Four Test Types by Employee Category and Employer Type

The following series of graphs subdivide the preceding test type/employee category rates by employer type. Two graphs, one for drugs and one for alcohol, are presented for the four test types combined and for each test type. They show the rates by employer type for each employee category. This series of graphs is followed by two tables that provide the statistical basis for the rates.

**Rates for Four Test Types Combined by Employee Category and Employer Type**

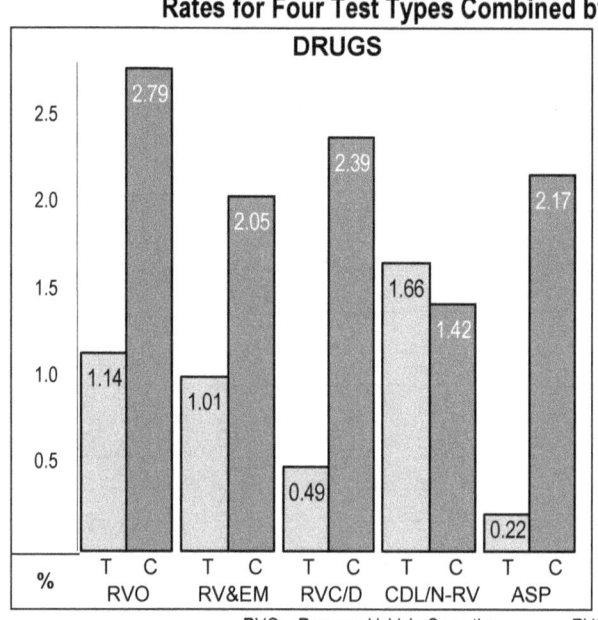

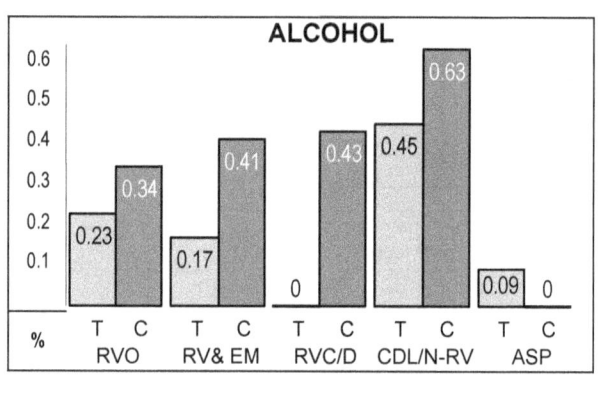

**Random Rates by Employee Category and Employer Type**

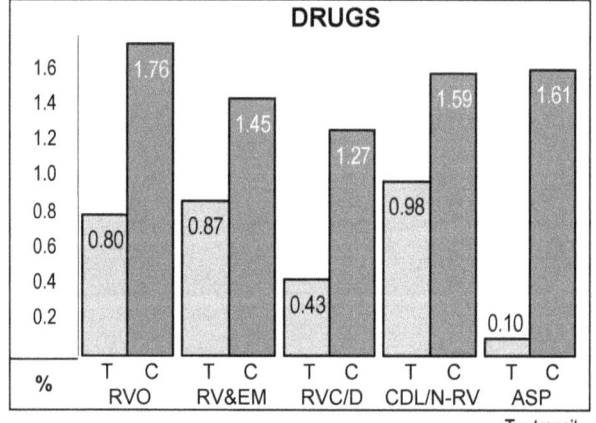

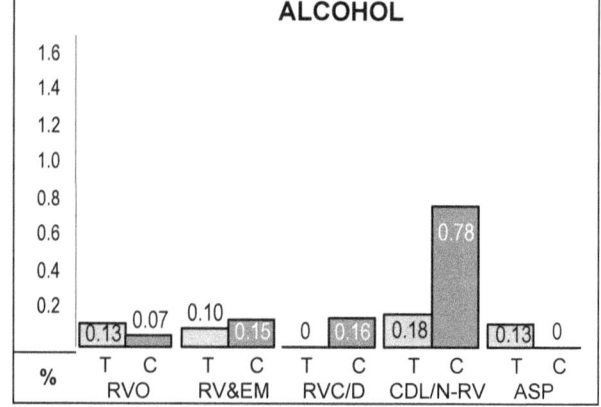

*The following graphs do not contain columns for employee categories that show a rate of "0" in the test type/employee category graphs on page 4-8. Some of the rates in two of those graphs are presented on a separate scale because their sample sizes are too small to be representative of their populations.*

## Post-Accident Rates by Employee Category and Employer Type

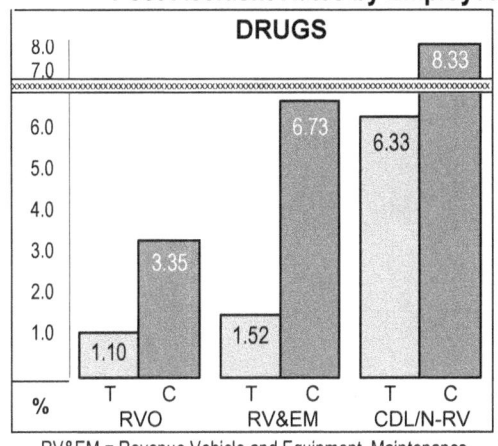

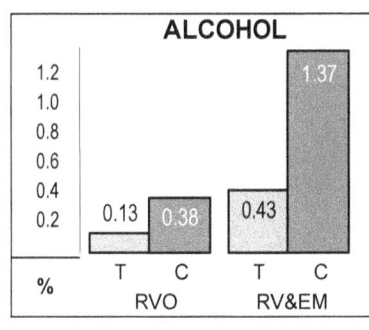

T = transit    C = contractor
RVO = Revenue Vehicle Operation
RV&EM = Revenue Vehicle and Equipment Maintenance    CDL/N-RV = CDL/Non-Revenue Vehicle

## Reasonable Suspicion Rates by Employee Category and Employer Type

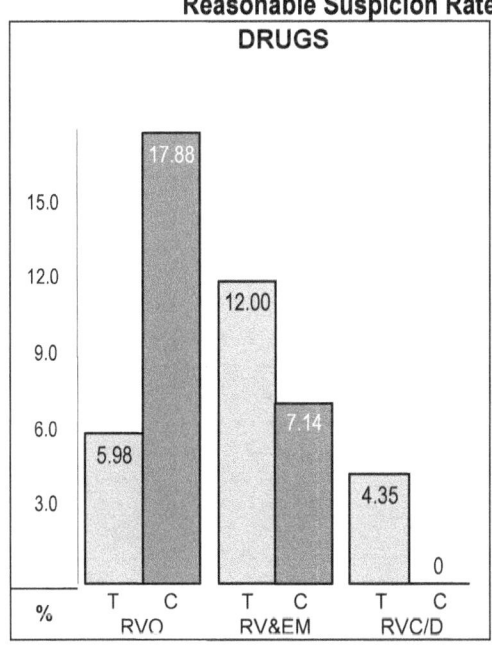

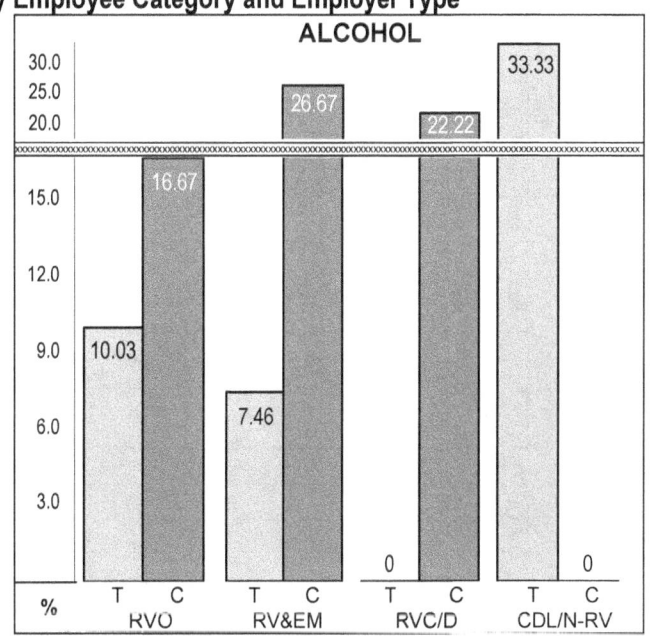

T = transit    C = contractor
RVO = Revenue Vehicle Operation    RV&EM = Revenue Vehicle and Equipment Maintenance
RVC/D = Revenue Vehicle Control/Dispatching    CDL/N-RV = CDL/Non-Revenue Vehicle

## Pre-Employment Rates by Employee Category and Employer Type

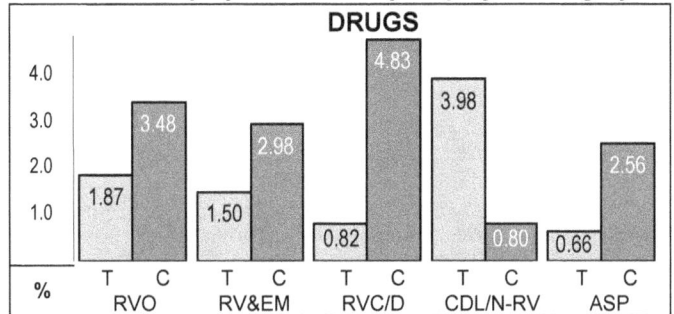

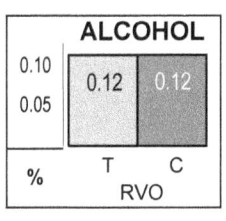

T = transit    C = contractor
RVO = Revenue Vehicle Operation    RV&EM = Revenue Vehicle and Equipment Maintenance
RVC/D = Revenue Vehicle Control/Dispatching    CDL/N-RV = CDL/Non-Revenue Vehicle    ASP = Armed Security Personnel

## Tests, Positives, and Refusals by Test Type, Employee Category, and Employer Type

| | | Drugs | | | | | | | | | |
|---|---|---|---|---|---|---|---|---|---|---|---|
| | | Random | | Post-Accident | | Reasonable Suspicion | | Pre-Employment | | Total | |
| | | Transit | Contractor | Transit | Contractor | Transit | Contractor | Transit | Contractor | Transit | Contractor |
| RVO | TE | 72,705 | 19,791 | 10,003 | 2,780 | 368 | 151 | 31,060 | 23,876 | 114,136 | 46,598 |
| | R+P | 583 | 349 | 110 | 93 | 22 | 27 | 582 | 831 | 1,297 | 1,300 |
| | P | 528 | 315 | 104 | 81 | 20 | 26 | 558 | 781 | 1,210 | 1,203 |
| | TR | 55 | 34 | 6 | 12 | 2 | 1 | 24 | 50 | 87 | 97 |
| | RTT | 34 | 21 | 3 | 11 | 1 | 1 | 16 | 31 | 54 | 64 |
| | SB | 17 | 5 | 1 | 1 | 1 | 0 | 2 | 1 | 21 | 7 |
| | Adul | 2 | 8 | 0 | 0 | 0 | 0 | 3 | 10 | 5 | 18 |
| | Sub | 2 | 0 | 2 | 0 | 0 | 0 | 3 | 8 | 7 | 8 |
| | R Rate | 0.076 | 0.172 | 0.060 | 0.432 | 0.543 | 0.662 | 0.077 | 0.209 | 0.076 | 0.208 |
| RV&EM | TE | 23,256 | 4,346 | 526 | 104 | 75 | 14 | 4,054 | 2,217 | 27,911 | 6,681 |
| | R+P | 203 | 63 | 8 | 7 | 9 | 1 | 61 | 66 | 281 | 137 |
| | P | 187 | 53 | 6 | 7 | 8 | 1 | 61 | 61 | 262 | 122 |
| | TR | 16 | 10 | 2 | 0 | 1 | 0 | 0 | 5 | 19 | 15 |
| | RTT | 10 | 9 | 2 | 0 | 1 | 0 | 0 | 4 | 13 | 13 |
| | SB | 1 | 1 | 0 | 0 | 0 | 0 | 0 | 1 | 1 | 2 |
| | Adul | 3 | 0 | 0 | 0 | 0 | 0 | 0 | 0 | 3 | 0 |
| | Sub | 2 | 0 | 0 | 0 | 0 | 0 | 0 | 0 | 2 | 0 |
| | R Rate | 0.069 | 0.230 | 0.380 | 0 | 1.333 | 0 | 0 | 0.226 | 0.068 | 0.225 |
| RVC/D | TE | 7,471 | 2,044 | 81 | 26 | 23 | 5 | 1,223 | 974 | 8,798 | 3,049 |
| | R+P | 32 | 26 | 0 | 0 | 1 | 0 | 10 | 47 | 43 | 73 |
| | P | 28 | 22 | 0 | 0 | 0 | 0 | 10 | 43 | 38 | 65 |
| | TR | 4 | 4 | 0 | 0 | 1 | 0 | 0 | 4 | 5 | 8 |
| | RTT | 3 | 2 | 0 | 0 | 1 | 0 | 0 | 3 | 4 | 5 |
| | SB | 0 | 1 | 0 | 0 | 0 | 0 | 0 | 0 | 0 | 1 |
| | Adul | 1 | 1 | 0 | 0 | 0 | 0 | 0 | 1 | 1 | 2 |
| | Sub | 0 | 0 | 0 | 0 | 0 | 0 | 0 | 0 | 0 | 0 |
| | R Rate | 0.054 | 0.196 | 0 | 0 | 4.348 | 0 | 0 | 0.411 | 0.057 | 0.262 |
| CDL/N-RV | TE | 2,748 | 441 | 79 | 12 | 20 | 0 | 653 | 250 | 3,500 | 703 |
| | R+P | 27 | 7 | 5 | 1 | 0 | 0 | 26 | 2 | 58 | 10 |
| | P | 26 | 6 | 5 | 1 | 0 | 0 | 22 | 2 | 53 | 9 |
| | TR | 1 | 1 | 0 | 0 | 0 | 0 | 4 | 0 | 5 | 1 |
| | RTT | 0 | 0 | 0 | 0 | 0 | 0 | 3 | 0 | 3 | 0 |
| | SB | 1 | 1 | 0 | 0 | 0 | 0 | 0 | 0 | 1 | 1 |
| | Adul | 0 | 0 | 0 | 0 | 0 | 0 | 1 | 0 | 1 | 0 |
| | Sub | 0 | 0 | 0 | 0 | 0 | 0 | 0 | 0 | 0 | 0 |
| | R Rate | 0.036 | 0.227 | 0 | 0 | 0 | 0 | 0.613 | 0 | 0.143 | 0.142 |
| ASP | TE | 2,059 | 436 | 64 | 40 | 0 | 1 | 607 | 860 | 2,730 | 1,337 |
| | R+P | 2 | 7 | 0 | 0 | 0 | 0 | 4 | 22 | 6 | 29 |
| | P | 2 | 3 | 0 | 0 | 0 | 0 | 4 | 20 | 6 | 23 |
| | TR | 0 | 4 | 0 | 0 | 0 | 0 | 0 | 2 | 0 | 6 |
| | RTT | 0 | 4 | 0 | 0 | 0 | 0 | 0 | 2 | 0 | 6 |
| | SB | 0 | 0 | 0 | 0 | 0 | 0 | 0 | 0 | 0 | 0 |
| | Adul | 0 | 0 | 0 | 0 | 0 | 0 | 0 | 0 | 0 | 0 |
| | Sub | 0 | 0 | 0 | 0 | 0 | 0 | 0 | 0 | 0 | 0 |
| | R Rate | 0 | 0.917 | 0 | 0 | 0 | 0 | 0 | 0.233 | 0 | 0.449 |

RVO = Revenue Vehicle Operation          RV&EM = Revenue Vehicle and Equipment Maintenance
RVC/D = Revenue Vehicle Control/Dispatching          CDL/N-RV = CDL/Non-Revenue Vehicle          ASP = Armed Security Personnel
TE = testing events          P = positives          R = refusals          TR = total refusals          R Rate = refusal rate
RTT = refusal to take test          SB = shy bladder          Adul = adulterated          Sub = substituted

## Tests, Positives, and Refusals by Test Type, Employee Category, and Employer Type

| | | Alcohol | | | | | | | | | |
|---|---|---|---|---|---|---|---|---|---|---|---|
| | | Random | | Post-Accident | | Reasonable Suspicion | | Pre-Employment | | Total | |
| | | Transit | Contractor | Transit | Contractor | Transit | Contractor | Transit | Contractor | Transit | Contractor |
| RVO | TE | 23,022 | 5,680 | 9,376 | 2,343 | 359 | 132 | 5,082 | 2,589 | 37,839 | 10,744 |
| | R+P | 30 | 4 | 12 | 9 | 36 | 22 | 6 | 3 | 84 | 38 |
| | P | 22 | 2 | 8 | 2 | 36 | 20 | 5 | 3 | 71 | 27 |
| | TR | 8 | 2 | 4 | 7 | 0 | 2 | 1 | 0 | 13 | 11 |
| | RTT | 5 | 2 | 2 | 7 | 0 | 2 | 0 | 0 | 7 | 11 |
| | SL | 3 | 0 | 2 | 0 | 0 | 0 | 1 | 0 | 6 | 0 |
| | R Rate | 0.035 | 0.035 | 0.043 | 0.299 | 0.000 | 1.515 | 0.020 | 0 | 0.034 | 0.102 |
| RV&EM | TE | 7,288 | 1,299 | 466 | 73 | 67 | 15 | 937 | 183 | 8,758 | 1,570 |
| | R+P | 7 | 2 | 2 | 1 | 5 | 4 | 0 | 0 | 14 | 7 |
| | P | 7 | 2 | 0 | 0 | 4 | 3 | 0 | 0 | 11 | 5 |
| | TR | 0 | 0 | 2 | 1 | 1 | 1 | 0 | 0 | 3 | 2 |
| | RTT | 0 | 0 | 1 | 1 | 1 | 1 | 0 | 0 | 2 | 2 |
| | SL | 0 | 0 | 1 | 0 | 0 | 0 | 0 | 0 | 1 | 0 |
| | R Rate | 0 | 0 | 0.429 | 1.370 | 1.493 | 6.667 | 0 | 0 | 0.034 | 0.127 |
| RVC/D | TE | 2,252 | 630 | 67 | 22 | 24 | 9 | 214 | 71 | 2,557 | 732 |
| | R+P | 0 | 1 | 0 | 0 | 0 | 2 | 0 | 0 | 0 | 3 |
| | P | 0 | 0 | 0 | 0 | 0 | 1 | 0 | 0 | 0 | 1 |
| | TR | 0 | 1 | 0 | 0 | 0 | 1 | 0 | 0 | 0 | 2 |
| | RTT | 0 | 1 | 0 | 0 | 0 | 1 | 0 | 0 | 0 | 2 |
| | SL | 0 | 0 | 0 | 0 | 0 | 0 | 0 | 0 | 0 | 0 |
| | R Rate | 0 | 0.159 | 0 | 0 | 0 | 11.111 | 0 | 0 | 0 | 0.273 |
| CDL/N-RV | TE | 1,125 | 129 | 74 | 5 | 12 | 2 | 132 | 22 | 1,343 | 158 |
| | R+P | 2 | 1 | 0 | 0 | 4 | 0 | 0 | 0 | 6 | 1 |
| | P | 2 | 1 | 0 | 0 | 4 | 0 | 0 | 0 | 6 | 1 |
| | TR | 0 | 0 | 0 | 0 | 0 | 0 | 0 | 0 | 0 | 0 |
| | RTT | 0 | 0 | 0 | 0 | 0 | 0 | 0 | 0 | 0 | 0 |
| | SL | 0 | 0 | 0 | 0 | 0 | 0 | 0 | 0 | 0 | 0 |
| | R Rate | 0 | 0 | 0 | 0 | 0 | 0 | 0 | 0 | 0 | 0 |
| ASP | TE | 759 | 133 | 55 | 9 | 0 | 0 | 285 | 157 | 1,099 | 299 |
| | R+P | 1 | 0 | 0 | 0 | 0 | 0 | 0 | 0 | 1 | 0 |
| | P | 1 | 0 | 0 | 0 | 0 | 0 | 0 | 0 | 1 | 0 |
| | TR | 0 | 0 | 0 | 0 | 0 | 0 | 0 | 0 | 0 | 0 |
| | RTT | 0 | 0 | 0 | 0 | 0 | 0 | 0 | 0 | 0 | 0 |
| | SL | 0 | 0 | 0 | 0 | 0 | 0 | 0 | 0 | 0 | 0 |
| | R Rate | 0 | 0 | 0 | 0 | 0 | 0 | 0 | 0 | 0 | 0 |

RVO = Revenue Vehicle Operation    RV&EM = Revenue Vehicle and Equipment Maintenance
RVC/D = Revenue Vehicle Control/Dispatching    CDL/N-RV = CDL/Non-Revenue Vehicle    ASP = Armed Security Personnel
TE = testing events    P = positives    R = refusals    TR = total refusals    RTT = refusal to take test    SL - shy lung    R Rate = refusal rate

### 4.2.2 Data for Four Test Types by Employee Category and Employer Size

The following series of graphs subdivide the test type/employee category rates by employer size. Two graphs, one for drugs and one for alcohol, are presented for the four test types combined and for each test type. This series of graphs is followed by two tables that provide the statistical basis for the rates.

*These graphs do not contain columns for employee categories that show a rate of "0" in the test type/employee category graphs on page 4-8.*

## Rates for Four Test Types Combined by Employee Category and Employer Size

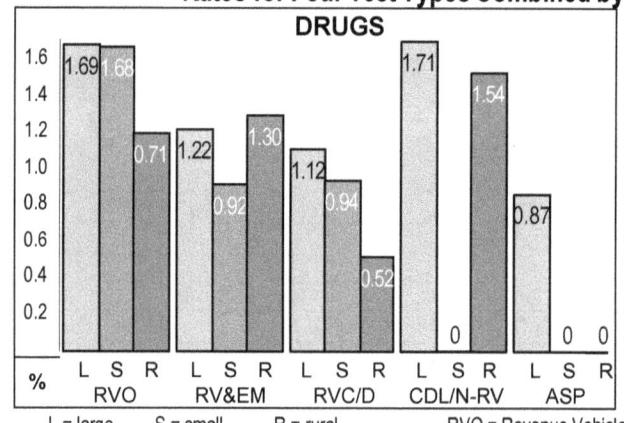

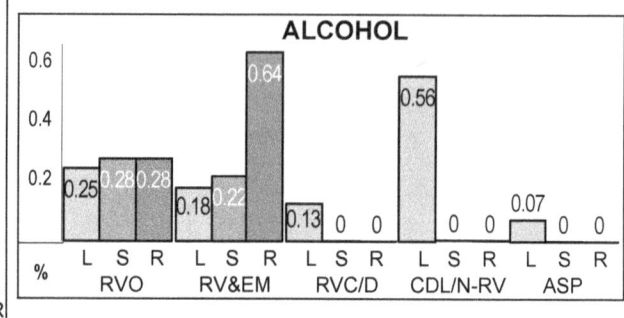

L = large    S = small    R = rural    RVO = Revenue Vehicle Operation    RV&EM = Revenue Vehicle and Equipment Maintenance
RVC/D = Revenue Vehicle Control/Dispatching    CDL/N-RV = CDL/Non-Revenue Vehicle    ASP = Armed Security Personnel

## Random Rates by Employee Category and Employer Size

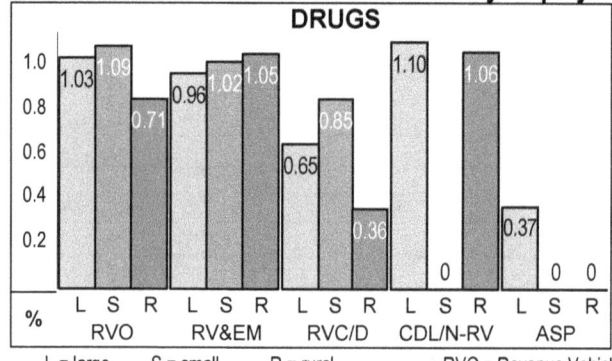

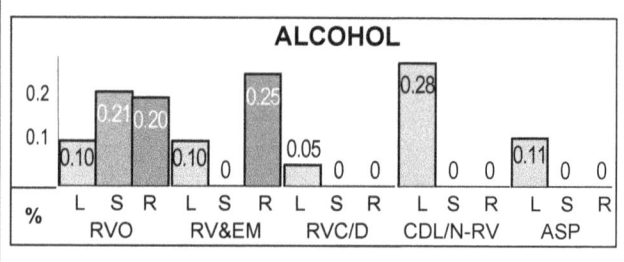

L = large    S = small    R = rural    RVO = Revenue Vehicle Operation    RV&EM = Revenue Vehicle and Equipment Maintenance
RVC/D = Revenue Vehicle Control/Dispatching    CDL/N-RV = CDL/Non-Revenue Vehicle    ASP = Armed Security Personnel

Two of the rates in the next drug graph are presented on a separate scale because their sample sizes are too small to be representative of their populations.

## Post-Accident Rates by Employee Category and Employer Size

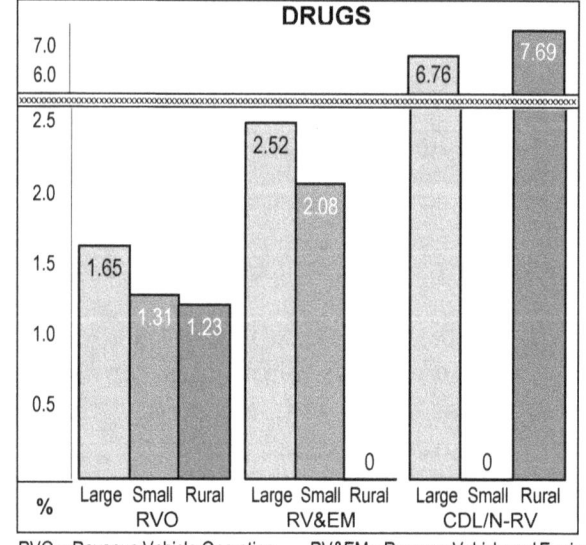

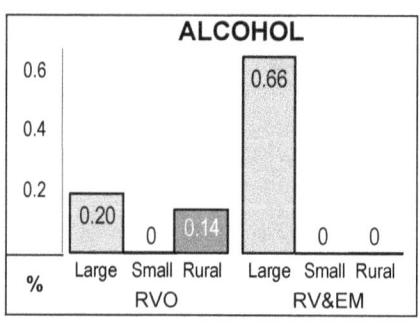

RVO = Revenue Vehicle Operation    RV&EM = Revenue Vehicle and Equipment Maintenance    CDL/N-RV = CDL/Non-Revenue Vehicle

Two of the rates in the next drug graph and two of the rates in the next alcohol graph are presented on a separate scale because their sample sizes are too small to be representative of their populations.

**Reasonable Suspicion Rates by Employee Category and Employer Size**

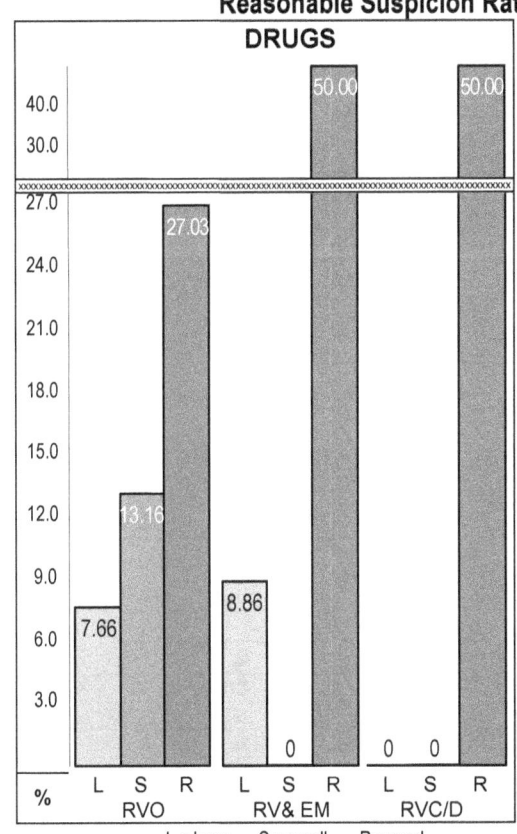

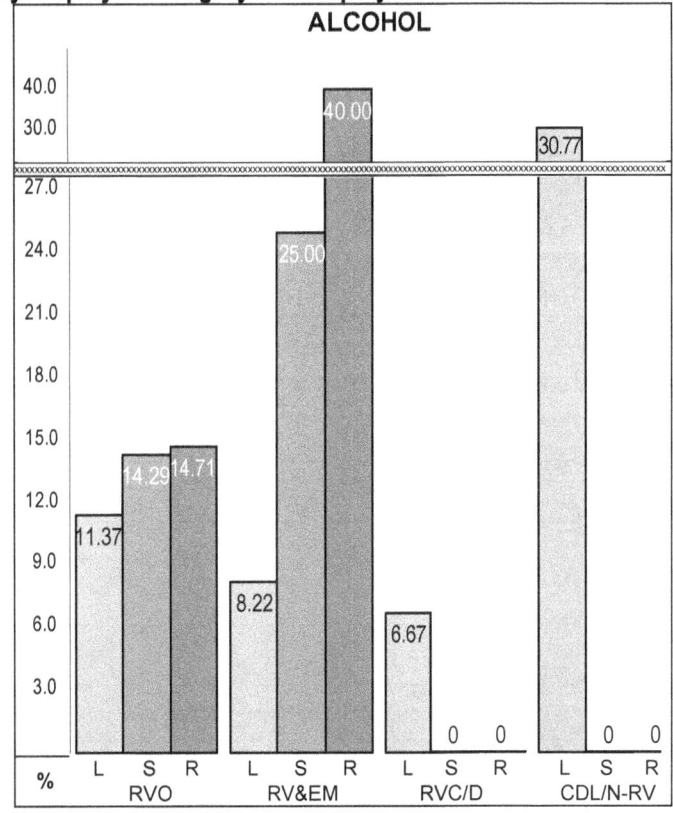

L = large    S = small    R = rural
RV&EM = Revenue Vehicle and Equipment Maintenance

RVO = Revenue Vehicle Operation
RVC/D = Revenue Vehicle Control/Dispatching    CDL/N-RV = CDL/Non-Revenue Vehicle

**Pre-Employment Rates by Employee Category and Employer Size**

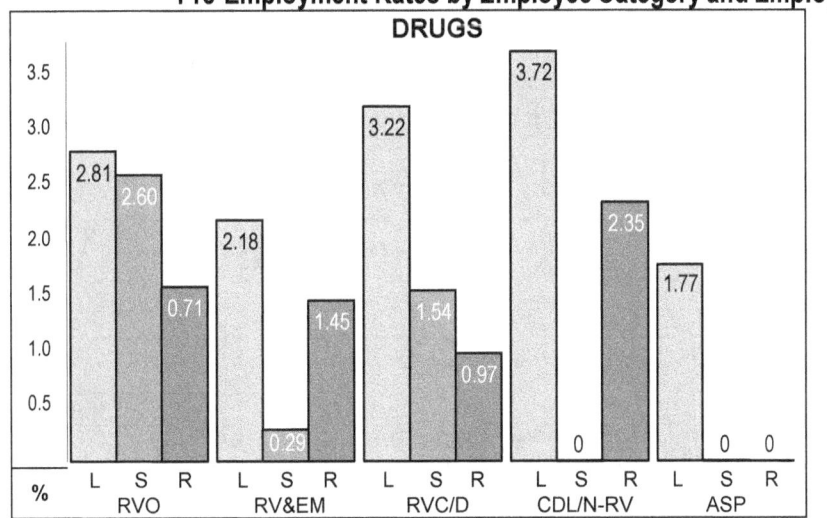

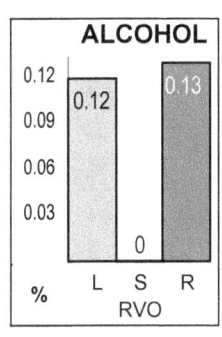

L = large    S = small    R = rural    RVO = Revenue Vehicle Operation    RV&EM = Revenue Vehicle and Equipment Maintenance
RVC/D = Revenue Vehicle Control/Dispatching    CDL/N-RV = CDL/Non-Revenue Vehicle    ASP = Armed Security Personnel

## Tests, Positives, and Refusals by Test Type, Employee Category, and Employer Size

| | | Random | | | Post-Accident | | | Reasonable Suspicion | | | Pre-Employment | | | Total | | |
|---|---|---|---|---|---|---|---|---|---|---|---|---|---|---|---|---|
| | | Large | Small | Rural | Large | Small | Rural | Large | Small | Rural | Large | Small | Rural | Large | Small | Rural |
| RVO | TE | 71,813 | 6,542 | 14,141 | 10,811 | 995 | 977 | 444 | 38 | 37 | 40,734 | 4,150 | 10,052 | 123,802 | 11,725 | 25,207 |
| | R+P | 741 | 71 | 120 | 178 | 13 | 12 | 34 | 5 | 10 | 1,145 | 108 | 160 | 2,098 | 197 | 302 |
| | P | 680 | 60 | 103 | 162 | 11 | 12 | 32 | 5 | 9 | 1,086 | 99 | 154 | 1,960 | 175 | 278 |
| | TR | 61 | 11 | 17 | 16 | 2 | 0 | 2 | 0 | 1 | 59 | 9 | 6 | 138 | 22 | 24 |
| | RTT | 35 | 5 | 15 | 12 | 2 | 0 | 1 | 0 | 1 | 39 | 5 | 3 | 87 | 12 | 19 |
| | SB | 14 | 6 | 2 | 2 | 0 | 0 | 1 | 0 | 0 | 1 | 1 | 1 | 18 | 7 | 3 |
| | Adul | 10 | 0 | 0 | 0 | 0 | 0 | 0 | 0 | 0 | 13 | 0 | 0 | 23 | 0 | 0 |
| | Sub | 2 | 0 | 0 | 2 | 0 | 0 | 0 | 0 | 0 | 6 | 3 | 2 | 10 | 3 | 2 |
| | R Rate | 0.085 | 0.168 | 0.120 | 0.148 | 0.201 | 0 | 0.450 | 0 | 2.703 | 0.145 | 0.217 | 0.060 | 0.111 | 0.188 | 0.095 |
| RV&EM | TE | 25,194 | 1,079 | 1,329 | 515 | 96 | 19 | 79 | 4 | 6 | 5,517 | 340 | 414 | 31,305 | 1,519 | 1,768 |
| | R+P | 241 | 11 | 14 | 13 | 2 | 0 | 7 | 0 | 3 | 120 | 1 | 6 | 381 | 14 | 23 |
| | P | 218 | 10 | 12 | 11 | 2 | 0 | 7 | 0 | 2 | 115 | 1 | 6 | 351 | 13 | 20 |
| | TR | 23 | 1 | 2 | 2 | 0 | 0 | 0 | 0 | 1 | 5 | 0 | 0 | 30 | 1 | 3 |
| | RTT | 17 | 1 | 1 | 2 | 0 | 0 | 0 | 0 | 1 | 4 | 0 | 0 | 23 | 1 | 2 |
| | SB | 2 | 0 | 0 | 0 | 0 | 0 | 0 | 0 | 0 | 1 | 0 | 0 | 3 | 0 | 0 |
| | Adul | 2 | 0 | 1 | 0 | 0 | 0 | 0 | 0 | 0 | 0 | 0 | 0 | 2 | 0 | 1 |
| | Sub | 2 | 0 | 0 | 0 | 0 | 0 | 0 | 0 | 0 | 0 | 0 | 0 | 2 | 0 | 0 |
| | R Rate | 0.091 | 0.093 | 0.150 | 0.388 | 0 | 0 | 0 | 0 | 16.667 | 0.091 | 0 | 0 | 0.096 | 0.066 | 0.170 |
| RVC/D | TE | 6,733 | 824 | 1,958 | 95 | 3 | 9 | 25 | 1 | 2 | 1,552 | 130 | 515 | 8,405 | 958 | 2,484 |
| | R+P | 44 | 7 | 7 | 0 | 0 | 0 | 0 | 0 | 1 | 50 | 2 | 5 | 94 | 9 | 13 |
| | P | 37 | 6 | 7 | 0 | 0 | 0 | 0 | 0 | 0 | 46 | 2 | 5 | 83 | 8 | 12 |
| | TR | 7 | 1 | 0 | 0 | 0 | 0 | 0 | 0 | 1 | 4 | 0 | 0 | 11 | 1 | 1 |
| | RTT | 4 | 1 | 0 | 0 | 0 | 0 | 0 | 0 | 1 | 3 | 0 | 0 | 7 | 1 | 1 |
| | SB | 1 | 0 | 0 | 0 | 0 | 0 | 0 | 0 | 0 | 0 | 0 | 0 | 1 | 0 | 0 |
| | Adul | 2 | 0 | 0 | 0 | 0 | 0 | 0 | 0 | 0 | 1 | 0 | 0 | 3 | 0 | 0 |
| | Sub | 0 | 0 | 0 | 0 | 0 | 0 | 0 | 0 | 0 | 0 | 0 | 0 | 0 | 0 | 0 |
| | R Rate | 0.104 | 0.121 | 0 | 0 | 0 | 0 | 0 | 0 | 50.00 | 0.258 | 0 | 0 | 0.131 | 0.104 | 0.040 |
| CDL/N-RV | TE | 2,539 | 82 | 568 | 74 | 4 | 13 | 10 | 0 | 10 | 592 | 56 | 255 | 3,215 | 142 | 846 |
| | R+P | 28 | 0 | 6 | 5 | 0 | 1 | 0 | 0 | 0 | 22 | 0 | 6 | 55 | 0 | 13 |
| | P | 27 | 0 | 5 | 5 | 0 | 1 | 0 | 0 | 0 | 19 | 0 | 5 | 51 | 0 | 11 |
| | TR | 1 | 0 | 1 | 0 | 0 | 0 | 0 | 0 | 0 | 3 | 0 | 1 | 4 | 0 | 2 |
| | RTT | 0 | 0 | 0 | 0 | 0 | 0 | 0 | 0 | 0 | 2 | 0 | 1 | 2 | 0 | 1 |
| | SB | 1 | 0 | 1 | 0 | 0 | 0 | 0 | 0 | 0 | 0 | 0 | 0 | 1 | 0 | 1 |
| | Adul | 0 | 0 | 0 | 0 | 0 | 0 | 0 | 0 | 0 | 1 | 0 | 0 | 1 | 0 | 0 |
| | Sub | 0 | 0 | 0 | 0 | 0 | 0 | 0 | 0 | 0 | 0 | 0 | 0 | 0 | 0 | 0 |
| | R Rate | 0.039 | 0 | 0.176 | 0 | 0 | 0 | 0 | 0 | 0 | 0.507 | 0.000 | 0.392 | 0.124 | 0 | 0.236 |
| ASP | TE | 2,456 | 29 | 10 | 97 | 6 | 1 | 1 | 0 | 0 | 1,465 | 2 | 0 | 4,019 | 37 | 11 |
| | R+P | 9 | 0 | 0 | 0 | 0 | 0 | 0 | 0 | 0 | 26 | 0 | 0 | 35 | 0 | 0 |
| | P | 5 | 0 | 0 | 0 | 0 | 0 | 0 | 0 | 0 | 24 | 0 | 0 | 29 | 0 | 0 |
| | TR | 4 | 0 | 0 | 0 | 0 | 0 | 0 | 0 | 0 | 2 | 0 | 0 | 6 | 0 | 0 |
| | RTT | 4 | 0 | 0 | 0 | 0 | 0 | 0 | 0 | 0 | 2 | 0 | 0 | 6 | 0 | 0 |
| | SB | 0 | 0 | 0 | 0 | 0 | 0 | 0 | 0 | 0 | 0 | 0 | 0 | 0 | 0 | 0 |
| | Adul | 0 | 0 | 0 | 0 | 0 | 0 | 0 | 0 | 0 | 0 | 0 | 0 | 0 | 0 | 0 |
| | Sub | 0 | 0 | 0 | 0 | 0 | 0 | 0 | 0 | 0 | 0 | 0 | 0 | 0 | 0 | 0 |
| | R Rate | 0.163 | 0 | 0 | 0 | 0 | 0 | 0 | 0 | 0 | 0.137 | 0 | 0 | 0.149 | 0 | 0 |

RVO = Revenue Vehicle Operation          RV&EM = Revenue Vehicle and Equipment Maintenance
RVC/D = Revenue Vehicle Control/Dispatching          CDL/N-RV = CDL/Non-Revenue Vehicle          ASP = Armed Security Personnel
TE = testing events          P = positives          R = refusals          TR = total refusals          R Rate = refusal rate
RTT = refusal to take test          SB - shy bladder          Adul = adulterated          Sub = substituted

**Tests, Positives, and Refusals by Test Type, Employee Category, and Employer Size**

| | | Alcohol | | | | | | | | | | | | | | |
|---|---|---|---|---|---|---|---|---|---|---|---|---|---|---|---|---|
| | | Random | | | Post-Accident | | | Reasonable Suspicion | | | Pre-Employment | | | Total | | |
| | | Large | Small | Rural | Large | Small | Rural | Large | Small | Rural | Large | Small | Rural | Large | Small | Rural |
| RVO | TE | 22,878 | 1,916 | 3,908 | 10,194 | 822 | 703 | 422 | 35 | 34 | 6,487 | 394 | 790 | 39,981 | 3,167 | 5,435 |
| | R+P | 22 | 4 | 8 | 20 | 0 | 1 | 48 | 5 | 5 | 8 | 0 | 1 | 98 | 9 | 15 |
| | P | 17 | 4 | 3 | 10 | 0 | 0 | 46 | 5 | 5 | 7 | 0 | 1 | 80 | 9 | 9 |
| | TR | 5 | 0 | 5 | 10 | 0 | 1 | 2 | 0 | 0 | 1 | 0 | 0 | 18 | 0 | 6 |
| | RTT | 3 | 0 | 4 | 9 | 0 | 0 | 2 | 0 | 0 | 0 | 0 | 0 | 14 | 0 | 4 |
| | SL | 2 | 0 | 1 | 1 | 0 | 0 | 0 | 0 | 0 | 1 | 0 | 0 | 4 | 0 | 2 |
| | R Rate | 0.022 | 0 | 0.128 | 0.098 | 0 | 0.142 | 0.474 | 0 | 0 | 0.015 | 0 | 0 | 0.045 | 0 | 0.110 |
| RV&EM | TE | 7,861 | 325 | 401 | 452 | 71 | 16 | 73 | 4 | 5 | 1,028 | 45 | 47 | 9,414 | 445 | 469 |
| | R+P | 8 | 0 | 1 | 3 | 0 | 0 | 6 | 1 | 2 | 0 | 0 | 0 | 17 | 1 | 3 |
| | P | 8 | 0 | 1 | 0 | 0 | 0 | 5 | 1 | 1 | 0 | 0 | 0 | 13 | 1 | 2 |
| | TR | 0 | 0 | 0 | 3 | 0 | 0 | 1 | 0 | 1 | 0 | 0 | 0 | 4 | 0 | 1 |
| | RTT | 0 | 0 | 0 | 2 | 0 | 0 | 1 | 0 | 1 | 0 | 0 | 0 | 3 | 0 | 1 |
| | SL | 0 | 0 | 0 | 1 | 0 | 0 | 0 | 0 | 0 | 0 | 0 | 0 | 1 | 0 | 0 |
| | R Rate | 0 | 0 | 0 | 0.664 | 0 | 0 | 1.370 | 0 | 20.00 | 0 | 0 | 0 | 0.042 | 0.000 | 0.213 |
| RVC/D | TE | 2,023 | 251 | 608 | 76 | 3 | 10 | 30 | 1 | 2 | 215 | 13 | 57 | 2,344 | 268 | 677 |
| | R+P | 1 | 0 | 0 | 0 | 0 | 0 | 2 | 0 | 0 | 0 | 0 | 0 | 3 | 0 | 0 |
| | P | 0 | 0 | 0 | 0 | 0 | 0 | 1 | 0 | 0 | 0 | 0 | 0 | 1 | 0 | 0 |
| | TR | 1 | 0 | 0 | 0 | 0 | 0 | 1 | 0 | 0 | 0 | 0 | 0 | 2 | 0 | 0 |
| | RTT | 1 | 0 | 0 | 0 | 0 | 0 | 1 | 0 | 0 | 0 | 0 | 0 | 2 | 0 | 0 |
| | SL | 0 | 0 | 0 | 0 | 0 | 0 | 0 | 0 | 0 | 0 | 0 | 0 | 0 | 0 | 0 |
| | R Rate | 0.049 | 0 | 0 | 0 | 0 | 0 | 3.333 | 0 | 0 | 0 | 0 | 0 | 0.085 | 0 | 0 |
| CDL/N-RV | TE | 1,054 | 30 | 170 | 67 | 3 | 9 | 13 | 0 | 1 | 118 | 4 | 32 | 1,252 | 37 | 212 |
| | R+P | 3 | 0 | 0 | 0 | 0 | 0 | 4 | 0 | 0 | 0 | 0 | 0 | 7 | 0 | 0 |
| | P | 3 | 0 | 0 | 0 | 0 | 0 | 4 | 0 | 0 | 0 | 0 | 0 | 7 | 0 | 0 |
| | TR | 0 | 0 | 0 | 0 | 0 | 0 | 0 | 0 | 0 | 0 | 0 | 0 | 0 | 0 | 0 |
| | RTT | 0 | 0 | 0 | 0 | 0 | 0 | 0 | 0 | 0 | 0 | 0 | 0 | 0 | 0 | 0 |
| | SL | 0 | 0 | 0 | 0 | 0 | 0 | 0 | 0 | 0 | 0 | 0 | 0 | 0 | 0 | 0 |
| | R Rate | 0 | 0 | 0 | 0 | 0 | 0 | 0 | 0 | 0 | 0 | 0 | 0 | 0 | 0 | 0 |
| ASP | TE | 883 | 8 | 1 | 64 | 0 | 0 | 0 | 0 | 0 | 442 | 0 | 0 | 1,389 | 8 | 1 |
| | R+P | 1 | 0 | 0 | 0 | 0 | 0 | 0 | 0 | 0 | 0 | 0 | 0 | 1 | 0 | 0 |
| | P | 1 | 0 | 0 | 0 | 0 | 0 | 0 | 0 | 0 | 0 | 0 | 0 | 1 | 0 | 0 |
| | TR | 0 | 0 | 0 | 0 | 0 | 0 | 0 | 0 | 0 | 0 | 0 | 0 | 0 | 0 | 0 |
| | RTT | 0 | 0 | 0 | 0 | 0 | 0 | 0 | 0 | 0 | 0 | 0 | 0 | 0 | 0 | 0 |
| | SL | 0 | 0 | 0 | 0 | 0 | 0 | 0 | 0 | 0 | 0 | 0 | 0 | 0 | 0 | 0 |
| | R Rate | 0 | 0 | 0 | 0 | 0 | 0 | 0 | 0 | 0 | 0 | 0 | 0 | 0 | 0 | 0 |

RVO = Revenue Vehicle Operation          RV&EM = Revenue Vehicle and Equipment Maintenance

RVC/D = Revenue Vehicle Control/Dispatching          CDL/N-RV = CDL/Non-Revenue Vehicle          ASP = Armed Security Personnel

TE = testing events          P = positives          R = refusals          TR = total refusals          RTT = refusal to take test          SL - shy lung          R Rate = refusal rate

## 4.3 Data for Four Test Types by FTA Region

The drug rates and alcohol rates for all four test types combined and random tests are shown by FTA region on the next four maps. The shading variations provide quick comparison. The exact rates are also included. The statistical basis for the rates is provided in the accompanying tables. The rates for post-accident, reasonable suspicion, and pre-employment tests appear in tables following the maps, along with the statistical basis for those rates. Data on the individual types of refusals follow the other data tables.  The data by region are subdivided by employer type and employer size in Sections 4.3.1 and 4.3.2, respectively.

### Drug Rates for Four Test Types Combined by FTA Region

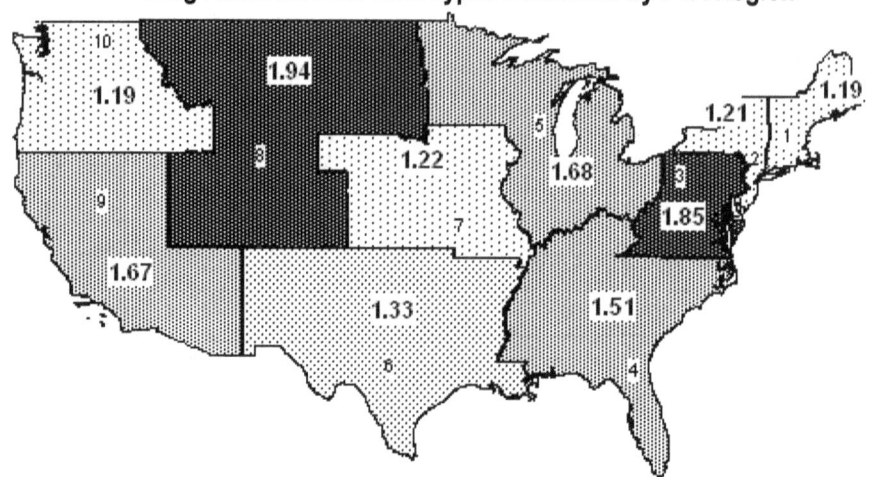

**Total Drug Tests, Positives, and Refusals for Four Test Types by Region**

| Region | Events | Positives | Refusals |
|---|---|---|---|
| 1 | 9,558 | 111 | 3 |
| 2 | 42,337 | 490 | 22 |
| 3 | 24,705 | 417 | 40 |
| 4 | 26,239 | 354 | 41 |
| 5 | 32,467 | 517 | 28 |
| 6 | 17,408 | 215 | 17 |
| 7 | 7,792 | 86 | 9 |
| 8 | 7,160 | 127 | 12 |
| 9 | 37,172 | 560 | 59 |
| 10 | 10,605 | 114 | 12 |

### Alcohol Rates for Four Test Types Combined by FTA Region

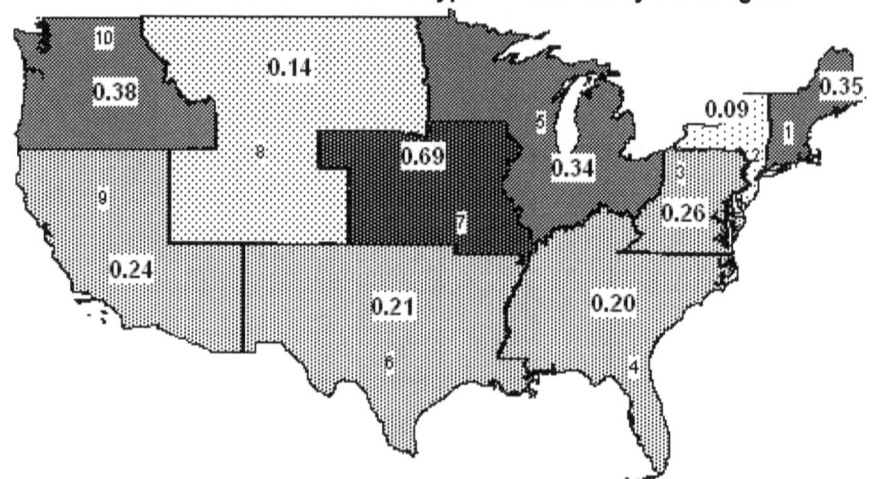

**Total Alcohol Tests, Positives, and Refusals for Four Test Types by Region**

| Region | Events | Positives | Refusals |
|---|---|---|---|
| 1 | 2,006 | 6 | 1 |
| 2 | 13,239 | 7 | 5 |
| 3 | 9,498 | 24 | 1 |
| 4 | 8,868 | 16 | 2 |
| 5 | 8,870 | 21 | 9 |
| 6 | 7,019 | 11 | 4 |
| 7 | 1,451 | 7 | 3 |
| 8 | 1,445 | 2 | 0 |
| 9 | 9,547 | 19 | 4 |
| 10 | 3,156 | 10 | 2 |

### Random Drug Rates by FTA Region

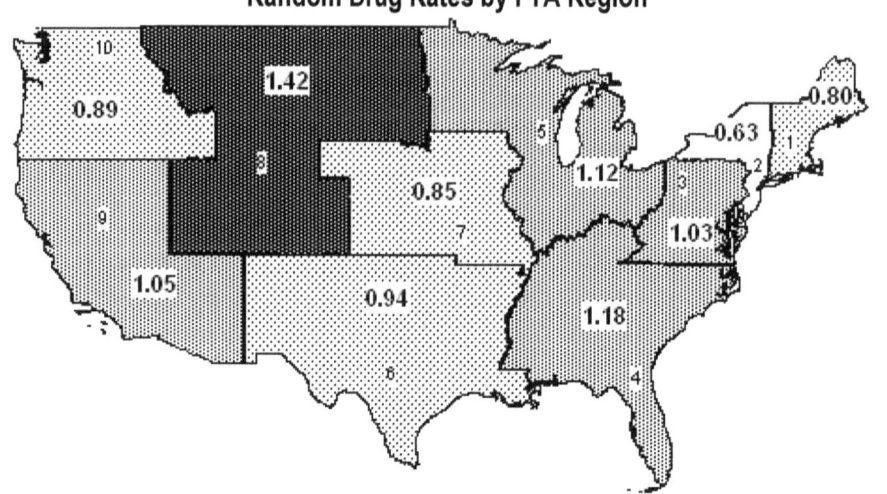

**Random Drug Tests, Positives, and Refusals by FTA Region**

| Region | Events | Positives | Refusals |
|---|---|---|---|
| 1 | 6,251 | 48 | 2 |
| 2 | 28,458 | 164 | 15 |
| 3 | 15,367 | 136 | 23 |
| 4 | 15,488 | 161 | 21 |
| 5 | 20,856 | 222 | 12 |
| 6 | 10,883 | 96 | 6 |
| 7 | 4,574 | 35 | 4 |
| 8 | 4,169 | 49 | 10 |
| 9 | 22,279 | 206 | 27 |
| 10 | 6,972 | 53 | 9 |

Events = testing events

## Random Alcohol Rates by FTA Region

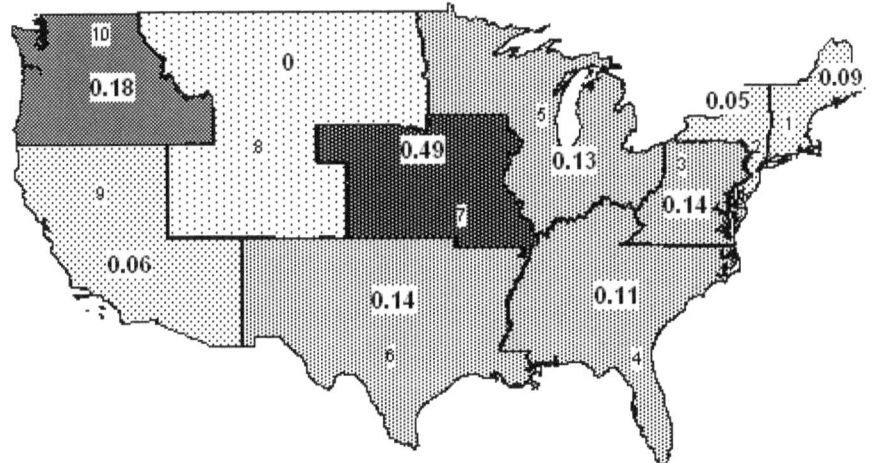

### Random Alcohol Tests, Positives, and Refusals by FTA Region

| Region | Testing Events | Positives | Refusals |
|---|---|---|---|
| 1 | 1,342 | 1 | 0 |
| 2 | 9,182 | 4 | 2 |
| 3 | 5,962 | 8 | 0 |
| 4 | 5,332 | 5 | 1 |
| 5 | 5,711 | 6 | 3 |
| 6 | 4,870 | 6 | 0 |
| 7 | 1,118 | 2 | 3 |
| 8 | 1,061 | 0 | 0 |
| 9 | 5,186 | 2 | 1 |
| 10 | 2,553 | 3 | 1 |

### Post-Accident Data by FTA Region

| Region | Drugs | | | | Alcohol | | | |
|---|---|---|---|---|---|---|---|---|
| | Testing Events | Positives | Refusals | Rate | Testing Events | Positives | Refusals | Rate |
| 1 | 435 | 7 | 1 | 1.84 | 396 | 0 | 1 | 0.25 |
| 2 | 1,930 | 20 | 2 | 1.14 | 1,840 | 1 | 3 | 0.22 |
| 3 | 1,153 | 32 | 1 | 2.86 | 1,022 | 0 | 0 | 0 |
| 4 | 2,501 | 28 | 1 | 1.16 | 2,223 | 2 | 1 | 0.13 |
| 5 | 2,489 | 40 | 8 | 1.93 | 2,362 | 1 | 6 | 0.30 |
| 6 | 1,296 | 13 | 2 | 1.16 | 1,103 | 0 | 1 | 0.09 |
| 7 | 351 | 6 | 0 | 1.71 | 299 | 2 | 0 | 0.67 |
| 8 | 338 | 11 | 0 | 3.25 | 276 | 1 | 0 | 0.36 |
| 9 | 2,693 | 45 | 5 | 1.86 | 2,470 | 3 | 1 | 0.16 |
| 10 | 529 | 2 | 0 | 0.38 | 499 | 0 | 1 | 0.20 |

### Reasonable Suspicion Data by FTA Region

| Region | Drugs | | | |
|---|---|---|---|---|
| | Testing Events | Positives | Refusals | Rate |
| 1 | 22 | 1 | 0 | 4.55 |
| 2 | 224 | 10 | 0 | 4.46 |
| 3 | 98 | 10 | 0 | 10.20 |
| 4 | 43 | 6 | 0 | 13.95 |
| 5 | 108 | 8 | 1 | 8.33 |
| 6 | 25 | 3 | 2 | 20.00 |
| 7 | 15 | 2 | 2 | 26.67 |
| 8 | 18 | 2 | 0 | 11.11 |
| 9 | 79 | 10 | 0 | 12.66 |
| 10 | 25 | 3 | 0 | 12.00 |

| Region | Alcohol | | | |
|---|---|---|---|---|
| | Testing Events | Positives | Refusals | Rate |
| 1 | 13 | 5 | 0 | 38.46 |
| 2 | 207 | 2 | 0 | 0.97 |
| 3 | 86 | 12 | 0 | 13.95 |
| 4 | 39 | 8 | 0 | 20.51 |
| 5 | 106 | 13 | 0 | 12.26 |
| 6 | 25 | 3 | 3 | 24.00 |
| 7 | 12 | 3 | 0 | 25.00 |
| 8 | 24 | 1 | 0 | 4.17 |
| 9 | 80 | 14 | 2 | 20.00 |
| 10 | 28 | 7 | 0 | 25.00 |

### Pre-Employment Data by FTA Region

| Region | Drugs | | | | Alcohol | | | |
|---|---|---|---|---|---|---|---|---|
| | Testing Events | Positives | Refusals | Rate | Testing Events | Positives | Refusals | Rate |
| 1 | 2,850 | 55 | 0 | 1.93 | 255 | 0 | 0 | 0 |
| 2 | 11,725 | 296 | 5 | 2.57 | 2,010 | 0 | 0 | 0 |
| 3 | 8,087 | 239 | 16 | 3.15 | 2,428 | 4 | 1 | 0.21 |
| 4 | 8,207 | 159 | 19 | 2.17 | 1,274 | 1 | 0 | 0.08 |
| 5 | 9,014 | 247 | 7 | 2.82 | 691 | 1 | 0 | 0.14 |
| 6 | 5,204 | 103 | 7 | 2.11 | 1,021 | 2 | 0 | 0.20 |
| 7 | 2,852 | 43 | 3 | 1.61 | 22 | 0 | 0 | 0 |
| 8 | 2,635 | 65 | 2 | 2.54 | 84 | 0 | 0 | 0 |
| 9 | 12,121 | 299 | 27 | 2.69 | 1,811 | 0 | 0 | 0 |
| 10 | 3,079 | 56 | 3 | 1.92 | 76 | 0 | 0 | 0 |

The total number of refusals by FTA Region listed in each of the preceding tables is subdivided by the individual types of refusals in the following table.

## Data on Refusal Types for Four Test Types by FTA Region

| | Drugs | | | | | | | | | | | | | | | | | | | Alcohol | | | | | | | | | |
|---|---|---|---|---|---|---|---|---|---|---|---|---|---|---|---|---|---|---|---|---|---|---|---|---|---|---|---|---|---|
| | Random | | | | Post-Accident | | | | Reasonable Suspicion | | | | Pre-Employment | | | | Total | | | | Random | | Post-Accident | | RS | | P-E | | Total | |
| Region | RTT | SB | Adul | Sub | RTT | SB | Adul | Sub | RTT | SB | Adul | Sub | RTT | SB | Adul | Sub | RTT | SB | Adul | Sub | RTT | SL | RTT | SL | RTT | SL | RTT | SL | RTT | SL |
| 1 | 2 | 0 | 0 | 0 | 1 | 0 | 0 | 0 | 0 | 0 | 0 | 0 | 0 | 0 | 0 | 0 | 3 | 0 | 0 | 0 | 0 | 0 | 1 | 0 | 0 | 0 | 0 | 0 | 1 | 0 |
| 2 | 6 | 4 | 4 | 1 | 2 | 0 | 0 | 0 | 0 | 0 | 0 | 0 | 3 | 0 | 1 | 1 | 11 | 4 | 5 | 2 | 2 | 0 | 2 | 1 | 0 | 0 | 0 | 0 | 4 | 1 |
| 3 | 17 | 4 | 1 | 1 | 1 | 0 | 0 | 0 | 0 | 0 | 0 | 0 | 16 | 0 | 0 | 0 | 34 | 4 | 1 | 1 | 0 | 0 | 0 | 0 | 0 | 0 | 0 | 1 | 0 | 1 |
| 4 | 10 | 10 | 0 | 1 | 1 | 0 | 0 | 0 | 0 | 0 | 0 | 0 | 14 | 2 | 1 | 2 | 25 | 12 | 1 | 3 | 1 | 0 | 1 | 0 | 0 | 0 | 0 | 0 | 2 | 0 |
| 5 | 9 | 1 | 1 | 1 | 7 | 0 | 0 | 1 | 0 | 1 | 0 | 0 | 1 | 0 | 1 | 5 | 17 | 2 | 2 | 7 | 1 | 2 | 5 | 1 | 0 | 0 | 0 | 0 | 6 | 3 |
| 6 | 6 | 0 | 0 | 0 | 0 | 1 | 0 | 1 | 2 | 0 | 0 | 0 | 5 | 0 | 0 | 2 | 13 | 1 | 0 | 3 | 0 | 0 | 1 | 0 | 3 | 0 | 0 | 0 | 4 | 0 |
| 7 | 3 | 1 | 0 | 0 | 0 | 0 | 0 | 0 | 2 | 0 | 0 | 0 | 3 | 0 | 0 | 0 | 8 | 1 | 0 | 0 | 2 | 1 | 0 | 0 | 0 | 0 | 0 | 0 | 2 | 1 |
| 8 | 8 | 2 | 0 | 0 | 0 | 0 | 0 | 0 | 0 | 0 | 0 | 0 | 1 | 0 | 0 | 1 | 9 | 2 | 0 | 1 | 0 | 0 | 0 | 0 | 0 | 0 | 0 | 0 | 0 | 0 |
| 9 | 14 | 4 | 9 | 0 | 4 | 1 | 0 | 0 | 0 | 0 | 0 | 0 | 14 | 1 | 12 | 0 | 32 | 6 | 21 | 0 | 1 | 0 | 1 | 0 | 2 | 0 | 0 | 0 | 4 | 0 |
| 10 | 8 | 1 | 0 | 0 | 0 | 0 | 0 | 0 | 0 | 0 | 0 | 0 | 2 | 1 | 0 | 0 | 10 | 2 | 0 | 0 | 1 | 0 | 0 | 1 | 0 | 0 | 0 | 0 | 1 | 1 |

RTT = refusal to take test    SB = shy bladder    SL = shy lung    Adul = adulterated    Sub = substituted

RS= Reasonable Suspicion    P-E – Pre-Employment

## 4.3.1 Data for Test Types by FTA Region and Employer Type

The drug rates and the alcohol rates by region for all four test types combined and for random tests are subdivided by employer type in the next four maps. The statistical basis for the rates for all four test types combined is provided in the table following the first pair of maps. The statistical basis for the random rates is provided in the table following the second pair of maps. That table is followed by three tables containing the rates by region and employer type for post-accident, reasonable suspicion, and pre-employment tests, respectively, along with the statistical basis for those rates. Data on the individual types of refusals follow the other data tables.

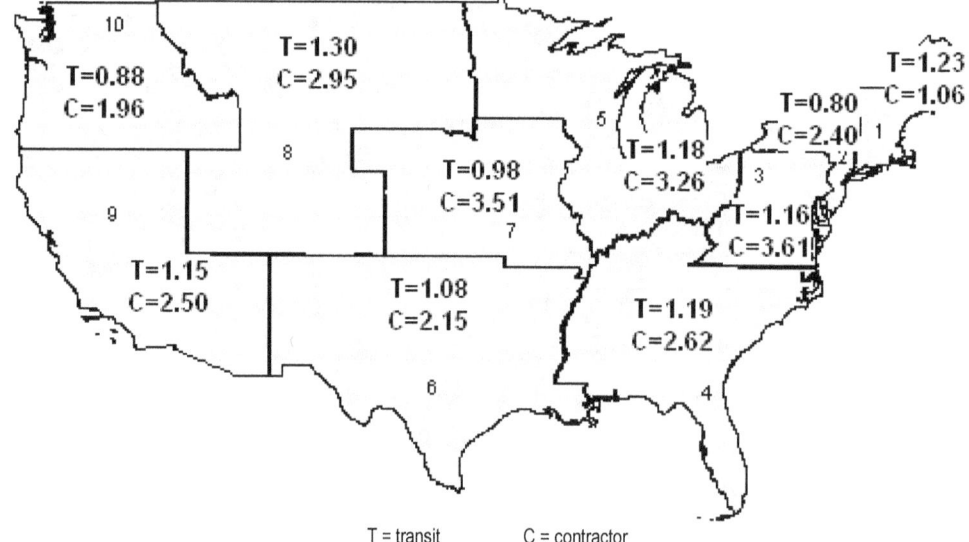

Drug Rates for Four Test Types Combined by FTA Region and Employer Type

T = transit    C = contractor

## Alcohol Rates for Four Test Types Combined by FTA Region and Employer Type

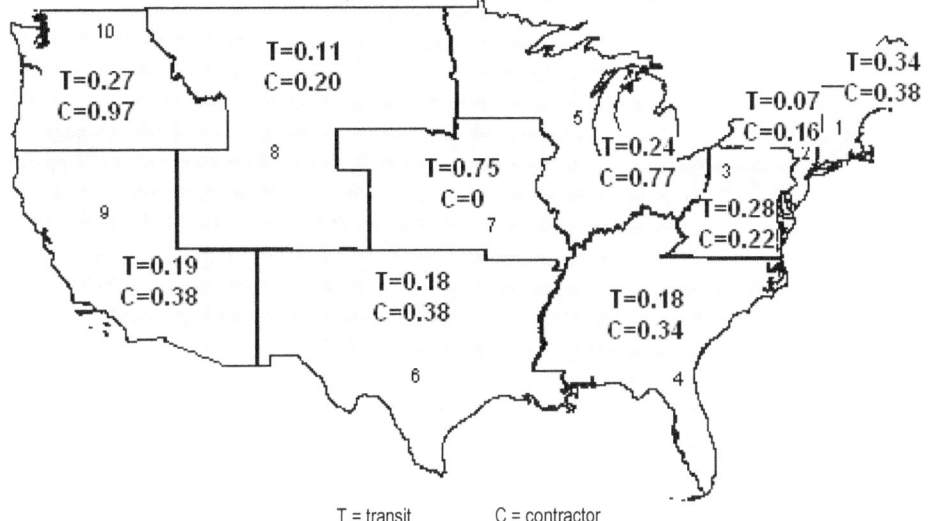

T = transit      C = contractor

## Total Tests, Positives, and Refusals for Four Test Types by FTA Region and Employer Type

| | Drugs | | | | | | Alcohol | | | | | |
|---|---|---|---|---|---|---|---|---|---|---|---|---|
| | Transit | | | Contractor | | | Transit | | | Contractor | | |
| Region | Testing Events | Positives | Refusals | Tests | Positives | Refusals | Testing Events | Positives | Refusals | Tests | Positives | Refusals |
| 1 | 7,389 | 90 | 1 | 2,169 | 21 | 2 | 1,482 | 5 | 0 | 524 | 1 | 1 |
| 2 | 31,523 | 238 | 15 | 10,814 | 252 | 7 | 10,173 | 5 | 2 | 3,066 | 2 | 3 |
| 3 | 17,744 | 187 | 19 | 6,961 | 230 | 21 | 7,228 | 19 | 1 | 2,270 | 5 | 0 |
| 4 | 20,444 | 221 | 22 | 5,795 | 133 | 19 | 7,706 | 13 | 1 | 1,162 | 3 | 1 |
| 5 | 24,687 | 274 | 17 | 7,780 | 243 | 11 | 7,189 | 12 | 5 | 1,681 | 9 | 4 |
| 6 | 13,265 | 133 | 10 | 4,143 | 82 | 7 | 5,965 | 10 | 1 | 1,054 | 1 | 3 |
| 7 | 7,052 | 64 | 5 | 740 | 22 | 4 | 1,336 | 7 | 3 | 115 | 0 | 0 |
| 8 | 4,385 | 51 | 6 | 2,775 | 76 | 6 | 944 | 1 | 0 | 501 | 1 | 0 |
| 9 | 23,045 | 249 | 17 | 14,127 | 311 | 42 | 6,935 | 12 | 1 | 2,612 | 7 | 3 |
| 10 | 7,541 | 62 | 4 | 3,064 | 52 | 8 | 2,638 | 5 | 2 | 518 | 5 | 0 |

## Random Drug Rates by FTA Region and Employer Type

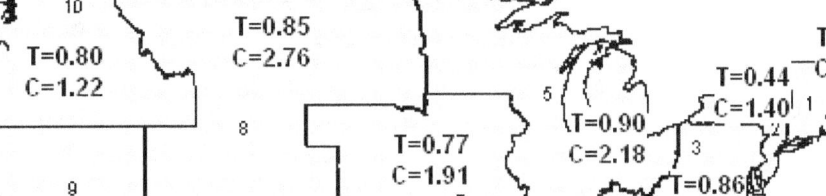

T = transit      C = contractor

## Random Alcohol Rates by FTA Region and Employer Type

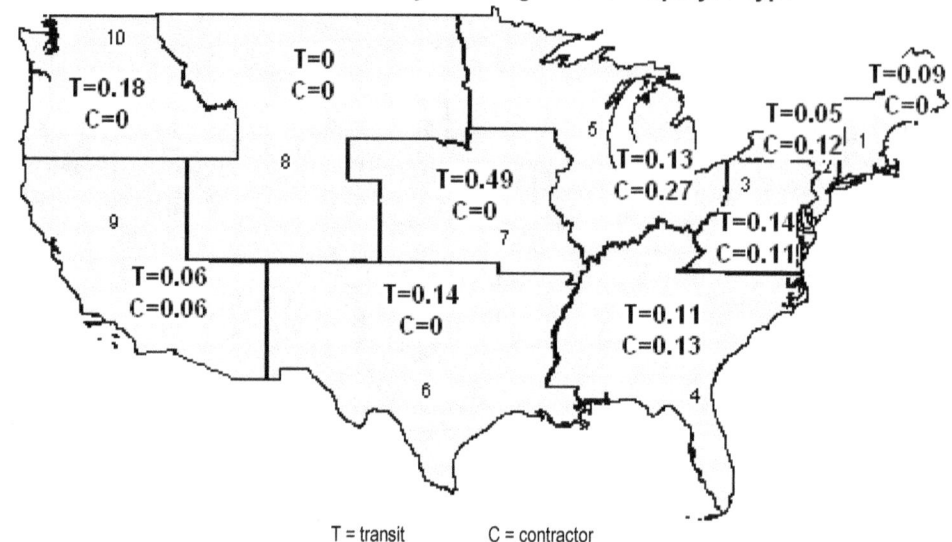

T = transit          C = contractor

## Random Tests, Positives, and Refusals by FTA Region and Employer Type

| | Drugs | | | | | | Alcohol | | | | | |
|---|---|---|---|---|---|---|---|---|---|---|---|---|
| | Transit | | | Contractor | | | Transit | | | Contractor | | |
| Region | Testing Events | Positives | Refusals | Testing Events | Positives | Refusals | Testing Events | Positives | Refusals | Testing Events | Positives | Refusals |
| 1 | 5,114 | 41 | 1 | 1,137 | 7 | 1 | 1,069 | 1 | 0 | 273 | 0 | 0 |
| 2 | 22,900 | 90 | 11 | 5,558 | 74 | 4 | 7,463 | 3 | 1 | 1,719 | 1 | 1 |
| 3 | 12,943 | 97 | 14 | 2,424 | 39 | 9 | 5,082 | 7 | 0 | 880 | 1 | 0 |
| 4 | 12,944 | 121 | 13 | 2,544 | 40 | 8 | 4,538 | 4 | 1 | 794 | 1 | 0 |
| 5 | 17,225 | 146 | 9 | 3,631 | 76 | 3 | 4,583 | 4 | 2 | 1,128 | 2 | 1 |
| 6 | 8,801 | 69 | 4 | 2,082 | 27 | 2 | 4,213 | 6 | 0 | 657 | 0 | 0 |
| 7 | 4,260 | 30 | 3 | 314 | 5 | 1 | 1,015 | 2 | 3 | 103 | 0 | 0 |
| 8 | 2,939 | 20 | 5 | 1,230 | 29 | 5 | 688 | 0 | 0 | 373 | 0 | 0 |
| 9 | 15,616 | 117 | 12 | 6,663 | 89 | 15 | 3,611 | 2 | 0 | 1,575 | 0 | 1 |
| 10 | 5,497 | 40 | 4 | 1,475 | 13 | 5 | 2,184 | 3 | 1 | 369 | 0 | 0 |

## Post-Accident Data by FTA Region and Employer Type

| | Drugs | | | | | | | | Alcohol | | | | | | | |
|---|---|---|---|---|---|---|---|---|---|---|---|---|---|---|---|---|
| | Transit | | | | Contractor | | | | Transit | | | | Contractor | | | |
| Region | TE | P | R | Rate | TE | P | R | Rate | TE | P | R | Rate | TE | P | R | Rate |
| 1 | 344 | 5 | 0 | 1.45 | 91 | 2 | 1 | 3.30 | 316 | 0 | 0 | 0 | 80 | 0 | 1 | 1.25 |
| 2 | 1,434 | 9 | 1 | 0.70 | 496 | 11 | 1 | 2.42 | 1,392 | 1 | 1 | 0.14 | 448 | 0 | 2 | 0.45 |
| 3 | 882 | 13 | 0 | 1.47 | 271 | 19 | 1 | 7.38 | 820 | 0 | 0 | 0 | 202 | 0 | 0 | 0.00 |
| 4 | 2,183 | 19 | 0 | 0.87 | 318 | 9 | 1 | 3.14 | 1,973 | 1 | 0 | 0.05 | 250 | 1 | 1 | 0.80 |
| 5 | 2,124 | 29 | 4 | 1.55 | 365 | 11 | 4 | 4.11 | 2,043 | 1 | 3 | 0.20 | 319 | 0 | 3 | 0.94 |
| 6 | 1,035 | 8 | 2 | 0.97 | 261 | 5 | 0 | 1.92 | 910 | 0 | 0 | 0 | 193 | 0 | 1 | 0.52 |
| 7 | 339 | 6 | 0 | 1.77 | 12 | 0 | 0 | 0 | 290 | 2 | 0 | 0.69 | 9 | 0 | 0 | 0 |
| 8 | 217 | 5 | 0 | 2.30 | 121 | 6 | 0 | 4.96 | 170 | 1 | 0 | 0.59 | 106 | 0 | 0 | 0 |
| 9 | 1,764 | 20 | 1 | 1.19 | 929 | 25 | 4 | 3.12 | 1,716 | 2 | 1 | 0.17 | 754 | 1 | 0 | 0.13 |
| 10 | 431 | 1 | 0 | 0.23 | 98 | 1 | 0 | 1.02 | 408 | 0 | 1 | 0.25 | 91 | 0 | 0 | 0 |

TE = testing events          P = positives          R = refusals

## Reasonable Suspicion Data by FTA Region and Employer Type

| | Drugs | | | | | | | | Alcohol | | | | | | | |
|---|---|---|---|---|---|---|---|---|---|---|---|---|---|---|---|---|
| | Transit | | | | Contractor | | | | Transit | | | | Contractor | | | |
| Region | TE | P | R | Rate | TE | P | R | Rate | TE | P | R | Rate | TE | P | R | Rate |
| 1 | 17 | 1 | 0 | 5.88 | 5 | 0 | 0 | 0 | 9 | 4 | 0 | 44.44 | 4 | 1 | 0 | 25.00 |
| 2 | 192 | 6 | 0 | 3.13 | 32 | 4 | 0 | 12.50 | 181 | 1 | 0 | 0.55 | 26 | 1 | 0 | 3.85 |
| 3 | 69 | 3 | 0 | 4.35 | 29 | 7 | 0 | 24.14 | 65 | 10 | 0 | 15.38 | 21 | 2 | 0 | 9.52 |
| 4 | 31 | 4 | 0 | 12.90 | 12 | 2 | 0 | 16.67 | 34 | 7 | 0 | 20.59 | 5 | 1 | 0 | 20.00 |
| 5 | 85 | 4 | 1 | 5.88 | 23 | 4 | 0 | 17.39 | 77 | 7 | 0 | 9.09 | 29 | 6 | 0 | 20.69 |
| 6 | 17 | 2 | 1 | 17.65 | 8 | 1 | 1 | 25.00 | 17 | 2 | 1 | 17.65 | 8 | 1 | 2 | 37.50 |
| 7 | 14 | 1 | 2 | 21.43 | 1 | 1 | 0 | 100.00 | 12 | 3 | 0 | 25.00 | 0 | 0 | 0 | 0 |
| 8 | 8 | 0 | 0 | 0 | 10 | 2 | 0 | 20.00 | 10 | 0 | 0 | 0 | 14 | 1 | 0 | 7.14 |
| 9 | 42 | 6 | 0 | 14.29 | 37 | 4 | 0 | 10.81 | 44 | 8 | 0 | 18.18 | 36 | 6 | 2 | 22.22 |
| 10 | 11 | 1 | 0 | 9.09 | 14 | 2 | 0 | 14.29 | 13 | 2 | 0 | 15.38 | 15 | 5 | 0 | 33.33 |

TE = testing events    P = positives    R = refusals

## Pre-Employment Data by FTA Region and Employer Type

| | Drugs | | | | | | | | Alcohol | | | | | | | |
|---|---|---|---|---|---|---|---|---|---|---|---|---|---|---|---|---|
| | Transit | | | | Contractor | | | | Transit | | | | Contractor | | | |
| Region | Tests | P | R | Rate | Tests | P | R | Rate | Tests | P | R | Rate | Tests | P | R | Rate |
| 1 | 1,914 | 43 | 0 | 2.25 | 936 | 12 | 0 | 1.28 | 88 | 0 | 0 | 0.00 | 167 | 0 | 0 | 0 |
| 2 | 6,997 | 133 | 3 | 1.94 | 4,728 | 163 | 2 | 3.49 | 1,137 | 0 | 0 | 0.00 | 873 | 0 | 0 | 0 |
| 3 | 3,850 | 74 | 5 | 2.05 | 4,237 | 165 | 11 | 4.15 | 1,261 | 2 | 1 | 0.24 | 1,167 | 2 | 0 | 0.17 |
| 4 | 5,286 | 77 | 9 | 1.63 | 2,921 | 82 | 10 | 3.15 | 1,161 | 1 | 0 | 0.09 | 113 | 0 | 0 | 0 |
| 5 | 5,253 | 95 | 3 | 1.87 | 3,761 | 152 | 4 | 4.15 | 486 | 0 | 0 | 0.00 | 205 | 1 | 0 | 0.49 |
| 6 | 3,412 | 54 | 3 | 1.67 | 1,792 | 49 | 4 | 2.96 | 825 | 2 | 0 | 0.24 | 196 | 0 | 0 | 0 |
| 7 | 2,439 | 27 | 0 | 1.11 | 413 | 16 | 3 | 4.60 | 19 | 0 | 0 | 0.00 | 3 | 0 | 0 | 0 |
| 8 | 1,221 | 26 | 1 | 2.21 | 1,414 | 39 | 1 | 2.83 | 76 | 0 | 0 | 0.00 | 8 | 0 | 0 | 0 |
| 9 | 5,623 | 106 | 4 | 1.96 | 6,498 | 193 | 23 | 3.32 | 1,564 | 0 | 0 | 0.00 | 247 | 0 | 0 | 0 |
| 10 | 1,602 | 20 | 0 | 1.25 | 1,477 | 36 | 3 | 2.64 | 33 | 0 | 0 | 0.00 | 43 | 0 | 0 | 0 |

TE = testing events    P = positives    R = refusals

## Data on Refusal Types for Four Test Types by FTA Region and Employer Type

| | Drugs | | | | | | | | | | | | | | | | | | | | | | | | | | | | | | | | | | | | | | | |
|---|---|---|---|---|---|---|---|---|---|---|---|---|---|---|---|---|---|---|---|---|---|---|---|---|---|---|---|---|---|---|---|---|---|---|---|---|---|---|---|---|
| | Random | | | | | | | | Post-Accident | | | | | | | | Reasonable Suspicion | | | | | | | | Pre-Employment | | | | | | | | Total | | | | | | | |
| | Transit | | | | Contractor | | | | Transit | | | | Contractor | | | | Transit | | | | Contractor | | | | Transit | | | | Contractor | | | | Transit | | | | Contractor | | | |
| Region | RT | SB | A | S | RT | SB | A | S | RT | SB | A | S | RT | SB | A | S | RT | SB | A | S | RT | SB | A | S | RT | SB | A | S | RT | SB | A | S | RT | SB | A | S | RT | SB | A | S |
| 1 | 1 | 0 | 0 | 0 | 1 | 0 | 0 | 0 | 0 | 0 | 0 | 0 | 1 | 0 | 0 | 0 | 0 | 0 | 0 | 0 | 0 | 0 | 0 | 0 | 0 | 0 | 0 | 0 | 0 | 0 | 0 | 0 | 1 | 0 | 0 | 0 | 2 | 0 | 0 | 0 |
| 2 | 4 | 4 | 2 | 1 | 2 | 0 | 2 | 0 | 1 | 0 | 0 | 0 | 1 | 0 | 0 | 0 | 0 | 0 | 0 | 0 | 0 | 0 | 0 | 0 | 2 | 0 | 1 | 0 | 1 | 0 | 0 | 1 | 7 | 4 | 3 | 1 | 4 | 0 | 2 | 1 |
| 3 | 9 | 3 | 1 | 1 | 8 | 1 | 0 | 0 | 0 | 0 | 0 | 0 | 1 | 0 | 0 | 0 | 0 | 0 | 0 | 0 | 0 | 0 | 0 | 0 | 5 | 0 | 0 | 0 | 11 | 0 | 0 | 0 | 14 | 3 | 1 | 1 | 20 | 1 | 0 | 0 |
| 4 | 7 | 5 | 0 | 1 | 3 | 5 | 0 | 0 | 0 | 0 | 0 | 0 | 1 | 0 | 0 | 0 | 0 | 0 | 0 | 0 | 0 | 0 | 0 | 0 | 6 | 1 | 1 | 1 | 8 | 1 | 0 | 1 | 13 | 6 | 1 | 2 | 12 | 6 | 0 | 1 |
| 5 | 6 | 1 | 1 | 1 | 3 | 0 | 0 | 0 | 3 | 0 | 0 | 1 | 4 | 0 | 0 | 0 | 1 | 0 | 0 | 0 | 0 | 0 | 0 | 0 | 0 | 0 | 1 | 2 | 1 | 0 | 0 | 3 | 9 | 2 | 2 | 4 | 8 | 0 | 0 | 3 |
| 6 | 4 | 0 | 0 | 0 | 2 | 0 | 0 | 0 | 0 | 1 | 0 | 1 | 0 | 0 | 0 | 0 | 1 | 0 | 0 | 0 | 1 | 0 | 0 | 0 | 3 | 0 | 0 | 0 | 2 | 0 | 0 | 2 | 8 | 1 | 0 | 1 | 5 | 0 | 0 | 2 |
| 7 | 2 | 1 | 0 | 0 | 1 | 0 | 0 | 0 | 0 | 0 | 0 | 0 | 0 | 0 | 0 | 0 | 2 | 0 | 0 | 0 | 0 | 0 | 0 | 0 | 0 | 0 | 0 | 0 | 3 | 0 | 0 | 0 | 4 | 1 | 0 | 0 | 4 | 0 | 0 | 0 |
| 8 | 3 | 2 | 0 | 0 | 5 | 0 | 0 | 0 | 0 | 0 | 0 | 0 | 0 | 0 | 0 | 0 | 0 | 0 | 0 | 0 | 0 | 0 | 0 | 0 | 0 | 0 | 0 | 1 | 1 | 0 | 0 | 0 | 3 | 2 | 0 | 1 | 6 | 0 | 0 | 0 |
| 9 | 8 | 2 | 2 | 0 | 6 | 2 | 7 | 0 | 1 | 0 | 0 | 0 | 3 | 1 | 0 | 0 | 0 | 0 | 0 | 0 | 0 | 0 | 0 | 0 | 3 | 0 | 1 | 0 | 11 | 1 | 11 | 0 | 12 | 2 | 3 | 0 | 20 | 4 | 18 | 0 |
| 10 | 3 | 1 | 0 | 0 | 5 | 0 | 0 | 0 | 0 | 0 | 0 | 0 | 0 | 0 | 0 | 0 | 0 | 0 | 0 | 0 | 0 | 0 | 0 | 0 | 0 | 0 | 0 | 0 | 2 | 1 | 0 | 0 | 3 | 1 | 0 | 0 | 7 | 1 | 0 | 0 |

RT = refusal to take test    SB = shy bladder    A = adulterated    S = substituted

### Data on Refusal Types for Four Test Types by FTA Region and Employer Type

| | Alcohol | | | | | | | | | | | | | | | | | | | |
|---|---|---|---|---|---|---|---|---|---|---|---|---|---|---|---|---|---|---|---|---|
| | Random | | | | Post-Accident | | | | Reasonable Suspicion | | | | Pre-Employment | | | | Total | | | |
| | Transit | | Contractor | | Transit | | Contractor | | Transit | | Contractor | | Transit | | Contractor | | Transit | | Contractor | |
| Region | RTT | SL | RTT | SL | RTT | SL | RTT | SL | RTT | SL | RTT | SL | RTT | SL | RTT | SL | RTT | SL | RTT | SL |
| 1 | 0 | 0 | 0 | 0 | 0 | 0 | 1 | 0 | 0 | 0 | 0 | 0 | 0 | 0 | 0 | 0 | 0 | 0 | 1 | 0 |
| 2 | 1 | 0 | 1 | 0 | 0 | 1 | 2 | 0 | 0 | 0 | 0 | 0 | 0 | 0 | 0 | 0 | 1 | 1 | 3 | 0 |
| 3 | 0 | 0 | 0 | 0 | 0 | 0 | 0 | 0 | 0 | 0 | 0 | 0 | 0 | 1 | 0 | 0 | 0 | 1 | 0 | 0 |
| 4 | 1 | 0 | 0 | 0 | 0 | 0 | 1 | 0 | 0 | 0 | 0 | 0 | 0 | 0 | 0 | 0 | 1 | 0 | 1 | 0 |
| 5 | 0 | 2 | 1 | 0 | 2 | 1 | 3 | 0 | 0 | 0 | 0 | 0 | 0 | 0 | 0 | 0 | 2 | 3 | 4 | 0 |
| 6 | 0 | 0 | 0 | 0 | 0 | 0 | 1 | 0 | 1 | 0 | 2 | 0 | 0 | 0 | 0 | 0 | 1 | 0 | 3 | 0 |
| 7 | 2 | 1 | 0 | 0 | 0 | 0 | 0 | 0 | 0 | 0 | 0 | 0 | 0 | 0 | 0 | 0 | 2 | 1 | 0 | 0 |
| 8 | 0 | 0 | 0 | 0 | 0 | 0 | 0 | 0 | 0 | 0 | 0 | 0 | 0 | 0 | 0 | 0 | 0 | 0 | 0 | 0 |
| 9 | 0 | 0 | 1 | 0 | 1 | 0 | 0 | 0 | 0 | 0 | 2 | 0 | 0 | 0 | 0 | 0 | 1 | 0 | 3 | 0 |
| 10 | 1 | 0 | 0 | 0 | 0 | 1 | 1 | 0 | 0 | 0 | 0 | 0 | 0 | 0 | 0 | 0 | 1 | 1 | 1 | 0 |

RTT = refusal to take test          SL = shy lung

## 4.3.2 Data for Four Test Types by FTA Region and Employer Size

The drug rates and the alcohol rates by region for all four test types combined and for random tests are subdivided by large employer in the following four maps. The shading variations provide quick comparison. The exact rates are also included. The statistical basis for the rates is provided in the accompanying tables. The rates by region and small and rural employers for the four test types combined appear in the table following the first pair of maps, along with the statistical basis for those rates. The rates by region and small and rural employers for random tests appear in the table following the second pair of maps, along with the statistical basis for those rates. That table is followed by three pairs of tables containing the rates by region and all employer size categories for post-accident, reasonable suspicion, and pre-employment tests, respectively, along with the statistical basis for those rates. Data on the individual types of refusals follow the other data tables.

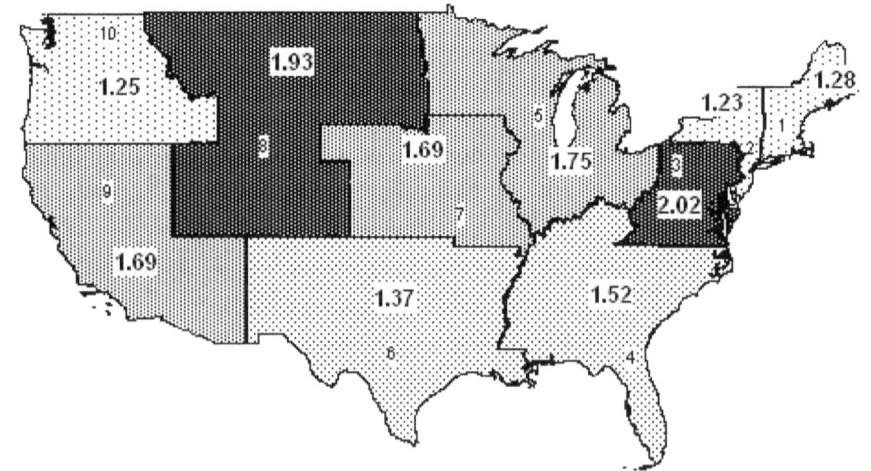

### Drug Rates for Four Test Types Combined by FTA Region and Employer Size—Large

### Total Drug Tests, Positives, and Refusals for Four Test Types by Region and Large Employer

| Region | Testing Events | Positives | Refusals |
|---|---|---|---|
| 1 | 5,800 | 72 | 2 |
| 2 | 41,012 | 482 | 22 |
| 3 | 21,349 | 395 | 36 |
| 4 | 16,428 | 225 | 24 |
| 5 | 24,907 | 415 | 20 |
| 6 | 12,703 | 163 | 11 |
| 7 | 3,197 | 49 | 5 |
| 8 | 4,764 | 86 | 6 |
| 9 | 32,516 | 496 | 53 |
| 10 | 8,070 | 91 | 10 |

## Alcohol Rates for Four Test Types Combined by FTA Region and Employer Size—Large

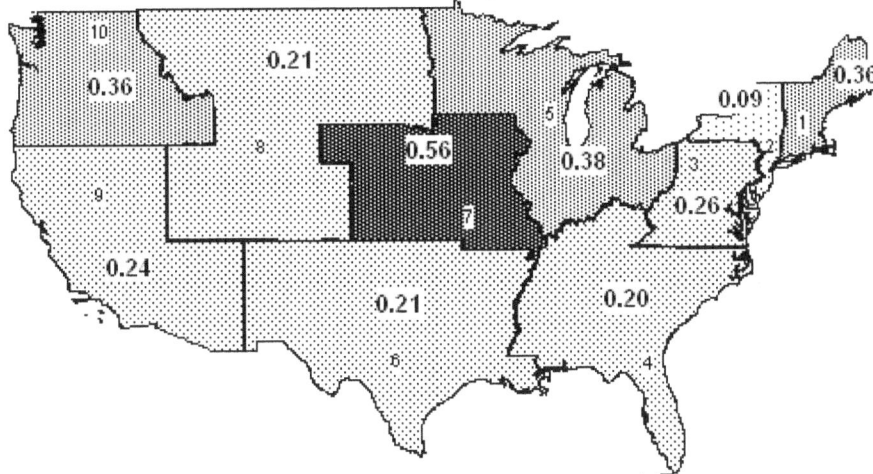

### Total Alcohol Tests, Positives, and Refusals for Four Test Types by Region and Large Employer

| Region | Testing Events | Positives | Refusals |
|---|---|---|---|
| 1 | 1,389 | 4 | 1 |
| 2 | 12,818 | 7 | 5 |
| 3 | 8,756 | 22 | 1 |
| 4 | 6,065 | 11 | 1 |
| 5 | 6,905 | 17 | 9 |
| 6 | 5,657 | 9 | 3 |
| 7 | 714 | 4 | 0 |
| 8 | 951 | 2 | 0 |
| 9 | 8,636 | 17 | 4 |
| 10 | 2,489 | 9 | 0 |

## Data for Four Test Types Combined by FTA Region and Employer Size—Small and Rural

| | Drugs | | | | | | | | Alcohol | | | | | | | |
|---|---|---|---|---|---|---|---|---|---|---|---|---|---|---|---|---|
| | Small | | | | Rural | | | | Small | | | | Rural | | | |
| Region | TE | P | R | Rate | TE | P | R | Rate | TE | P | R | Rate | TE | P | R | Rate |
| 1 | 1,222 | 6 | 1 | 0.57 | 216 | 1 | 0 | 0.46 | 2,536 | 33 | 0 | 1.30 | 401 | 1 | 0 | 0.25 |
| 2 | 295 | 1 | 0 | 0.34 | 161 | 0 | 0 | 0 | 1,030 | 7 | 0 | 0.68 | 260 | 0 | 0 | 0.00 |
| 3 | 1,236 | 4 | 1 | 0.40 | 285 | 1 | 0 | 0.35 | 2,120 | 18 | 3 | 0.99 | 457 | 1 | 0 | 0.22 |
| 4 | 2,780 | 57 | 10 | 2.41 | 964 | 2 | 0 | 0.21 | 7,031 | 72 | 7 | 1.12 | 1,839 | 3 | 1 | 0.22 |
| 5 | 3,364 | 46 | 4 | 1.49 | 905 | 3 | 0 | 0.33 | 4,196 | 56 | 4 | 1.43 | 1,060 | 1 | 0 | 0.09 |
| 6 | 1,135 | 14 | 0 | 1.23 | 370 | 2 | 0 | 0.54 | 3,570 | 38 | 6 | 1.23 | 992 | 0 | 1 | 0.10 |
| 7 | 618 | 7 | 0 | 1.13 | 142 | 1 | 0 | 0.70 | 3,977 | 30 | 4 | 0.85 | 595 | 2 | 3 | 0.84 |
| 8 | 983 | 22 | 2 | 2.44 | 242 | 0 | 0 | 0 | 1,413 | 19 | 4 | 1.63 | 252 | 0 | 0 | 0.00 |
| 9 | 1,789 | 29 | 5 | 1.90 | 284 | 0 | 0 | 0 | 2,867 | 35 | 1 | 1.26 | 627 | 2 | 0 | 0.32 |
| 10 | 959 | 10 | 1 | 1.15 | 356 | 0 | 0 | 0 | 1,576 | 13 | 1 | 0.89 | 311 | 1 | 2 | 0.96 |

TE = testing events    P = positives    R = refusals

## Random Drug Rates by FTA Region and Employer Size—Large

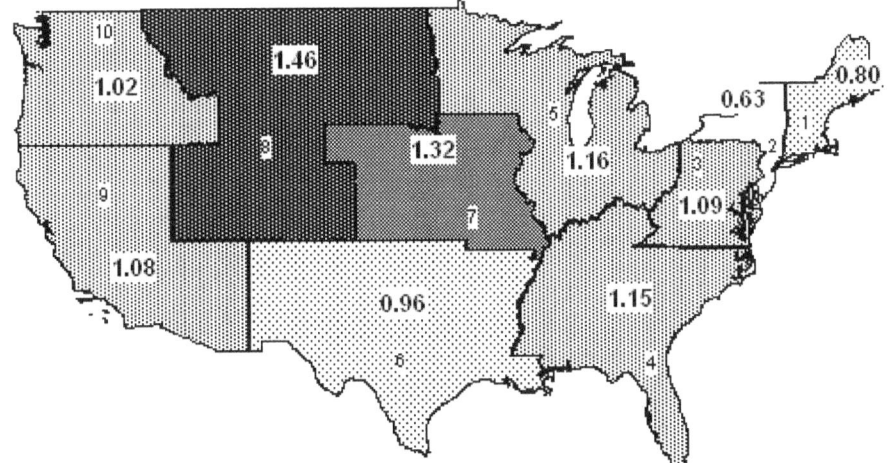

### Random Drug Tests, Positives, and Refusals by Region and Large Employer

| Region | Testing Events | Positives | Refusals |
|---|---|---|---|
| 1 | 3,991 | 31 | 1 |
| 2 | 27,585 | 160 | 15 |
| 3 | 13,152 | 124 | 20 |
| 4 | 9,965 | 102 | 13 |
| 5 | 15,983 | 178 | 7 |
| 6 | 8,327 | 77 | 3 |
| 7 | 1,816 | 22 | 2 |
| 8 | 2,806 | 36 | 5 |
| 9 | 19,698 | 189 | 23 |
| 10 | 5,412 | 48 | 7 |

## Random Alcohol Rates by FTA Region and Employer Size—Large

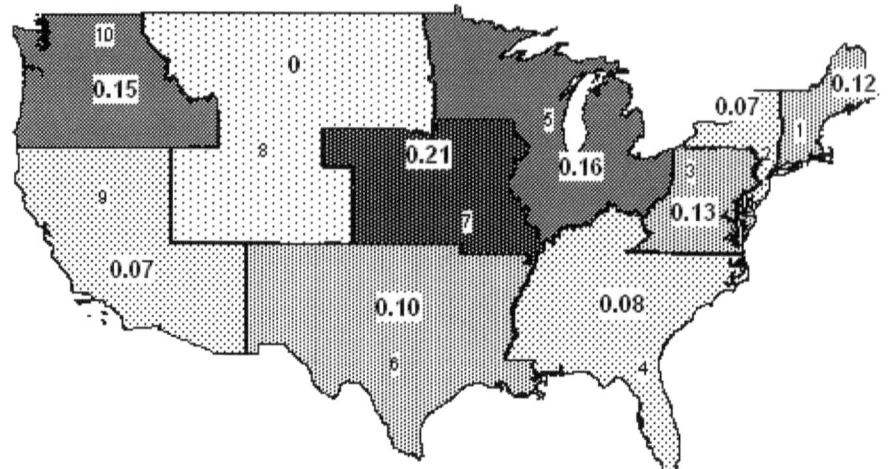

### Random Alcohol Tests, Positives, and Refusals by Region and Large Employer

| Region | Testing Events | Positives | Refusals |
|---|---|---|---|
| 1 | 836 | 1 | 0 |
| 2 | 8,887 | 4 | 2 |
| 3 | 5,383 | 7 | 0 |
| 4 | 3,540 | 3 | 0 |
| 5 | 4,370 | 4 | 3 |
| 6 | 3,933 | 4 | 0 |
| 7 | 474 | 1 | 0 |
| 8 | 720 | 0 | 0 |
| 9 | 4,547 | 2 | 1 |
| 10 | 2,009 | 3 | 0 |

## Random Test Data by FTA Region and Employer Size—Small and Rural

| | Drugs | | | | | | | | Alcohol | | | | | | | |
|---|---|---|---|---|---|---|---|---|---|---|---|---|---|---|---|---|
| | Small | | | | Rural | | | | Small | | | | Rural | | | |
| Region | TE | P | R | Rate | TE | P | R | Rate | TE | P | R | Rate | TE | P | R | Rate |
| 1 | 693 | 4 | 1 | 0.72 | 1,567 | 13 | 0 | 0.83 | 162 | 0 | 0 | 0.00 | 344 | 0 | 0 | 0.00 |
| 2 | 230 | 1 | 0 | 0.43 | 643 | 3 | 0 | 0.47 | 111 | 0 | 0 | 0.00 | 184 | 0 | 0 | 0.00 |
| 3 | 864 | 2 | 1 | 0.35 | 1,351 | 10 | 2 | 0.89 | 213 | 0 | 0 | 0.00 | 366 | 1 | 0 | 0.27 |
| 4 | 1,463 | 26 | 5 | 2.12 | 4,060 | 33 | 3 | 0.89 | 457 | 0 | 0 | 0.00 | 1,335 | 2 | 1 | 0.22 |
| 5 | 2,224 | 18 | 1 | 0.85 | 2,649 | 26 | 4 | 1.13 | 608 | 1 | 0 | 0.16 | 733 | 1 | 0 | 0.14 |
| 6 | 648 | 5 | 0 | 0.77 | 1,908 | 14 | 3 | 0.89 | 240 | 2 | 0 | 0.83 | 697 | 0 | 0 | 0.00 |
| 7 | 388 | 3 | 0 | 0.77 | 2,370 | 10 | 2 | 0.51 | 117 | 1 | 0 | 0.85 | 527 | 0 | 3 | 0.57 |
| 8 | 530 | 7 | 1 | 1.51 | 833 | 6 | 4 | 1.20 | 152 | 0 | 0 | 0.00 | 189 | 0 | 0 | 0.00 |
| 9 | 891 | 7 | 3 | 1.12 | 1,690 | 10 | 1 | 0.65 | 185 | 0 | 0 | 0.00 | 454 | 0 | 0 | 0.00 |
| 10 | 625 | 3 | 1 | 0.64 | 935 | 2 | 1 | 0.32 | 285 | 0 | 0 | 0.00 | 259 | 0 | 1 | 0.39 |

TE = testing events          P = positives          R = refusals

## Post-Accident Test Data by FTA Region and Employer Size

| | Drugs | | | | | | | | | | | |
|---|---|---|---|---|---|---|---|---|---|---|---|---|
| | Large | | | | Small | | | | Rural | | | |
| Region | Testing Events | Positives | Refusals | Rate | Testing Events | Positives | Refusals | Rate | Testing Events | Positives | Refusals | Rate |
| 1 | 341 | 6 | 1 | 2.05 | 42 | 0 | 0 | 0 | 52 | 1 | 0 | 1.92 |
| 2 | 1,883 | 20 | 2 | 1.17 | 13 | 0 | 0 | 0 | 34 | 0 | 0 | 0 |
| 3 | 1,013 | 30 | 1 | 3.06 | 80 | 0 | 0 | 0 | 60 | 2 | 0 | 3.33 |
| 4 | 1,832 | 21 | 0 | 1.15 | 389 | 3 | 1 | 1.03 | 280 | 4 | 0 | 1.43 |
| 5 | 2,102 | 35 | 7 | 2.00 | 233 | 3 | 1 | 1.72 | 154 | 2 | 0 | 1.30 |
| 6 | 981 | 9 | 2 | 1.12 | 118 | 3 | 0 | 2.54 | 197 | 1 | 0 | 0.51 |
| 7 | 257 | 6 | 0 | 2.33 | 28 | 0 | 0 | 0.00 | 66 | 0 | 0 | 0.00 |
| 8 | 226 | 6 | 0 | 2.65 | 61 | 2 | 0 | 3.28 | 51 | 3 | 0 | 5.88 |
| 9 | 2,505 | 44 | 5 | 1.96 | 96 | 1 | 0 | 1.04 | 92 | 0 | 0 | 0 |
| 10 | 452 | 1 | 0 | 0.22 | 44 | 1 | 0 | 2.27 | 33 | 0 | 0 | 0 |

## Post-Accident Test Data by FTA Region and Employer Size

| | Alcohol | | | | | | | | | | | |
|---|---|---|---|---|---|---|---|---|---|---|---|---|
| | Large | | | | Small | | | | Rural | | | |
| Region | Testing Events | Positives | Refusals | Rate | Testing Events | Positives | Refusals | Rate | Testing Events | Positives | Refusals | Rate |
| 1 | 323 | 0 | 1 | 0.31 | 32 | 0 | 0 | 0 | 41 | 0 | 0 | 0 |
| 2 | 1,799 | 1 | 3 | 0.22 | 11 | 0 | 0 | 0 | 30 | 0 | 0 | 0 |
| 3 | 910 | 0 | 0 | 0 | 69 | 0 | 0 | 0 | 43 | 0 | 0 | 0 |
| 4 | 1,652 | 2 | 1 | 0.18 | 364 | 0 | 0 | 0 | 207 | 0 | 0 | 0 |
| 5 | 2,049 | 1 | 6 | 0.34 | 188 | 0 | 0 | 0 | 125 | 0 | 0 | 0 |
| 6 | 879 | 0 | 1 | 0.11 | 88 | 0 | 0 | 0 | 136 | 0 | 0 | 0 |
| 7 | 231 | 2 | 0 | 0.87 | 21 | 0 | 0 | 0 | 47 | 0 | 0 | 0 |
| 8 | 211 | 1 | 0 | 0.47 | 36 | 0 | 0 | 0 | 29 | 0 | 0 | 0 |
| 9 | 2,349 | 3 | 1 | 0.17 | 59 | 0 | 0 | 0 | 62 | 0 | 0 | 0 |
| 10 | 450 | 0 | 0 | 0 | 31 | 0 | 0 | 0 | 18 | 0 | 1 | 5.56 |

## Reasonable Suspicion Test Data by FTA Region and Employer Size

| | Drugs | | | | | | | | | | | |
|---|---|---|---|---|---|---|---|---|---|---|---|---|
| | Large | | | | Small | | | | Rural | | | |
| Region | Testing Events | Positives | Refusals | Rate | Testing Events | Positives | Refusals | Rate | Testing Events | Positives | Refusals | Rate |
| 1 | 11 | 1 | 0 | 9.09 | 1 | 0 | 0 | 0 | 52 | 1 | 0 | 1.92 |
| 2 | 221 | 10 | 0 | 4.52 | 0 | 0 | 0 | 0 | 34 | 0 | 0 | 0 |
| 3 | 94 | 10 | 0 | 10.64 | 2 | 0 | 0 | 0 | 60 | 2 | 0 | 3.33 |
| 4 | 26 | 4 | 0 | 15.38 | 11 | 1 | 0 | 9.09 | 280 | 4 | 0 | 1.43 |
| 5 | 89 | 3 | 1 | 4.49 | 16 | 3 | 0 | 18.75 | 154 | 2 | 0 | 1.30 |
| 6 | 16 | 3 | 1 | 25.00 | 2 | 0 | 0 | 0 | 197 | 1 | 0 | 0.51 |
| 7 | 5 | 0 | 0 | 0 | 0 | 0 | 0 | 0 | 66 | 0 | 0 | 0 |
| 8 | 16 | 2 | 0 | 12.50 | 1 | 0 | 0 | 0 | 51 | 3 | 0 | 5.88 |
| 9 | 61 | 4 | 0 | 6.56 | 6 | 1 | 0 | 16.67 | 92 | 0 | 0 | 0 |
| 10 | 20 | 2 | 0 | 10.00 | 4 | 0 | 0 | 0 | 33 | 0 | 0 | 0 |

| | Alcohol | | | | | | | | | | | |
|---|---|---|---|---|---|---|---|---|---|---|---|---|
| | Large | | | | Small | | | | Rural | | | |
| Region | Testing Events | Positives | Refusals | Rate | Testing Events | Positives | Refusals | Rate | Testing Events | Positives | Refusals | Rate |
| 1 | 9 | 3 | 0 | 33.33 | 2 | 1 | 0 | 50.00 | 41 | 0 | 0 | 0 |
| 2 | 205 | 2 | 0 | 0.98 | 0 | 0 | 0 | 0 | 30 | 0 | 0 | 0 |
| 3 | 80 | 11 | 0 | 13.75 | 3 | 1 | 0 | 33.33 | 43 | 0 | 0 | 0 |
| 4 | 28 | 6 | 0 | 21.43 | 10 | 2 | 0 | 20.00 | 207 | 0 | 0 | 0 |
| 5 | 88 | 11 | 0 | 12.50 | 14 | 2 | 0 | 14.29 | 125 | 0 | 0 | 0 |
| 6 | 17 | 3 | 2 | 29.41 | 1 | 0 | 0 | 0 | 136 | 0 | 0 | 0 |
| 7 | 5 | 1 | 0 | 20.00 | 0 | 0 | 0 | 0 | 47 | 0 | 0 | 0 |
| 8 | 17 | 1 | 0 | 5.88 | 2 | 0 | 0 | 0 | 29 | 0 | 0 | 0 |
| 9 | 67 | 12 | 2 | 20.90 | 4 | 0 | 0 | 0 | 62 | 0 | 0 | 0 |
| 10 | 22 | 6 | 0 | 27.27 | 4 | 0 | 0 | 0 | 18 | 0 | 1 | 5.56 |

## Pre-Employment Test Data by FTA Region and Employer Size

### Drugs

| Region | Large Testing Events | Positives | Refusals | Rate | Small Testing Events | Positives | Refusals | Rate | Rural Testing Events | Positives | Refusals | Rate |
|---|---|---|---|---|---|---|---|---|---|---|---|---|
| 1 | 1,457 | 34 | 0 | 2.33 | 486 | 2 | 0 | 0.41 | 907 | 19 | 0 | 2.09 |
| 2 | 11,323 | 292 | 5 | 2.62 | 52 | 0 | 0 | 0.00 | 350 | 4 | 0 | 1.14 |
| 3 | 7,090 | 231 | 15 | 3.47 | 290 | 2 | 0 | 0.69 | 707 | 6 | 1 | 0.99 |
| 4 | 4,605 | 98 | 11 | 2.37 | 917 | 27 | 4 | 3.38 | 2,685 | 34 | 4 | 1.42 |
| 5 | 6,733 | 199 | 5 | 3.03 | 891 | 22 | 2 | 2.69 | 1,390 | 26 | 0 | 1.87 |
| 6 | 3,379 | 74 | 5 | 2.34 | 367 | 6 | 0 | 1.63 | 1,458 | 23 | 2 | 1.71 |
| 7 | 1,119 | 21 | 3 | 2.14 | 202 | 4 | 0 | 1.98 | 1,531 | 18 | 0 | 1.18 |
| 8 | 1,716 | 42 | 1 | 2.51 | 391 | 13 | 1 | 3.58 | 528 | 10 | 0 | 1.89 |
| 9 | 10,252 | 259 | 25 | 2.77 | 796 | 20 | 2 | 2.76 | 1,073 | 20 | 0 | 1.86 |
| 10 | 2,186 | 40 | 3 | 1.97 | 286 | 6 | 0 | 2.10 | 607 | 10 | 0 | 1.65 |

### Alcohol

| Region | Large Testing Events | Positives | Refusals | Rate | Small Testing Events | Positives | Refusals | Rate | Rural Testing Events | Positives | Refusals | Rate |
|---|---|---|---|---|---|---|---|---|---|---|---|---|
| 1 | 221 | 0 | 0 | 0 | 20 | 0 | 0 | 0 | 14 | 0 | 0 | 0 |
| 2 | 1,927 | 0 | 0 | 0 | 39 | 0 | 0 | 0 | 44 | 0 | 0 | 0 |
| 3 | 2,383 | 4 | 1 | 0.21 | 0 | 0 | 0 | 0 | 45 | 0 | 0 | 0 |
| 4 | 845 | 0 | 0 | 0 | 133 | 0 | 0 | 0 | 296 | 1 | 0 | 0.34 |
| 5 | 398 | 1 | 0 | 0.25 | 95 | 0 | 0 | 0 | 198 | 0 | 0 | 0 |
| 6 | 828 | 2 | 0 | 0.24 | 41 | 0 | 0 | 0 | 152 | 0 | 0 | 0 |
| 7 | 4 | 0 | 0 | 0 | 4 | 0 | 0 | 0 | 14 | 0 | 0 | 0 |
| 8 | 3 | 0 | 0 | 0 | 52 | 0 | 0 | 0 | 29 | 0 | 0 | 0 |
| 9 | 1,673 | 0 | 0 | 0 | 36 | 0 | 0 | 0 | 102 | 0 | 0 | 0 |
| 10 | 8 | 0 | 0 | 0 | 36 | 0 | 0 | 0 | 32 | 0 | 0 | 0 |

The next two tables subdivide the total number of refusals by region and employer size presented in the preceding tables by the individual types of refusals.

## Data on Refusal Types for Four Test Types by FTA Region and Employer Size

### Drugs

Column legend per cell group: R = refusal to take test, B = shy bladder, A = adulterated, S = substituted. Within each test type the three employer sizes (Large, Small, Rural) each list R, B, A, S.

| Region | Rnd Lg R | Rnd Lg B | Rnd Lg A | Rnd Lg S | Rnd Sm R | Rnd Sm B | Rnd Sm A | Rnd Sm S | Rnd Ru R | Rnd Ru B | Rnd Ru A | Rnd Ru S | PA Lg R | PA Lg B | PA Lg A | PA Lg S | PA Sm R | PA Sm B | PA Sm A | PA Sm S | PA Ru R | PA Ru B | PA Ru A | PA Ru S | RS Lg R | RS Lg B | RS Lg A | RS Lg S | RS Sm R | RS Sm B | RS Sm A | RS Sm S | RS Ru R | RS Ru B | RS Ru A | RS Ru S | PE Lg R | PE Lg B | PE Lg A | PE Lg S | PE Sm R | PE Sm B | PE Sm A | PE Sm S | PE Ru R | PE Ru B | PE Ru A | PE Ru S | Tot Lg R | Tot Lg B | Tot Lg A | Tot Lg S | Tot Sm R | Tot Sm B | Tot Sm A | Tot Sm S | Tot Ru R | Tot Ru B | Tot Ru A | Tot Ru S |
|---|---|---|---|---|---|---|---|---|---|---|---|---|---|---|---|---|---|---|---|---|---|---|---|---|---|---|---|---|---|---|---|---|---|---|---|---|---|---|---|---|---|---|---|---|---|---|---|---|---|---|---|---|---|---|---|---|---|---|---|---|
| 1 | 1 | 0 | 0 | 0 | 1 | 0 | 0 | 0 | 0 | 0 | 0 | 0 | 1 | 0 | 0 | 0 | 0 | 0 | 0 | 0 | 0 | 0 | 0 | 0 | 0 | 0 | 0 | 0 | 0 | 0 | 0 | 0 | 0 | 0 | 0 | 0 | 0 | 0 | 0 | 0 | 0 | 0 | 0 | 0 | 0 | 0 | 0 | 0 | 2 | 0 | 0 | 0 | 1 | 0 | 0 | 0 | 0 | 0 | 0 | 0 |
| 2 | 6 | 4 | 4 | 1 | 0 | 0 | 0 | 0 | 0 | 0 | 0 | 0 | 2 | 0 | 0 | 0 | 0 | 0 | 0 | 0 | 0 | 0 | 0 | 0 | 0 | 0 | 0 | 0 | 0 | 0 | 0 | 0 | 0 | 0 | 0 | 0 | 3 | 0 | 1 | 1 | 0 | 0 | 0 | 0 | 0 | 0 | 0 | 0 | 11 | 4 | 5 | 2 | 0 | 0 | 0 | 0 | 0 | 0 | 0 | 0 |
| 3 | 16 | 2 | 1 | 1 | 0 | 1 | 0 | 0 | 1 | 1 | 0 | 0 | 1 | 0 | 0 | 0 | 0 | 0 | 0 | 0 | 0 | 0 | 0 | 0 | 0 | 0 | 0 | 0 | 0 | 0 | 0 | 0 | 0 | 0 | 0 | 0 | 15 | 0 | 0 | 0 | 0 | 0 | 0 | 0 | 1 | 0 | 0 | 0 | 32 | 2 | 1 | 1 | 0 | 1 | 0 | 0 | 2 | 1 | 0 | 0 |
| 4 | 7 | 5 | 0 | 1 | 0 | 5 | 0 | 0 | 3 | 0 | 0 | 0 | 0 | 0 | 0 | 0 | 1 | 0 | 0 | 0 | 0 | 0 | 0 | 0 | 0 | 0 | 0 | 0 | 0 | 0 | 0 | 0 | 0 | 0 | 0 | 0 | 9 | 1 | 1 | 0 | 4 | 0 | 0 | 0 | 1 | 1 | 0 | 2 | 16 | 6 | 1 | 1 | 5 | 5 | 0 | 0 | 4 | 1 | 0 | 2 |
| 5 | 5 | 1 | 0 | 1 | 1 | 0 | 0 | 0 | 3 | 0 | 1 | 0 | 6 | 0 | 0 | 1 | 1 | 0 | 0 | 0 | 0 | 0 | 0 | 0 | 0 | 1 | 0 | 0 | 0 | 0 | 0 | 0 | 0 | 0 | 0 | 0 | 1 | 0 | 1 | 3 | 0 | 0 | 0 | 2 | 0 | 0 | 0 | 0 | 12 | 2 | 1 | 5 | 2 | 0 | 0 | 2 | 3 | 0 | 1 | 0 |
| 6 | 3 | 0 | 0 | 0 | 0 | 0 | 0 | 0 | 3 | 0 | 0 | 0 | 0 | 1 | 0 | 1 | 0 | 0 | 0 | 0 | 1 | 0 | 0 | 0 | 1 | 0 | 0 | 0 | 0 | 0 | 0 | 0 | 0 | 0 | 0 | 0 | 3 | 0 | 0 | 2 | 0 | 0 | 0 | 0 | 2 | 0 | 0 | 0 | 7 | 1 | 0 | 3 | 0 | 0 | 0 | 0 | 6 | 0 | 0 | 0 |
| 7 | 2 | 0 | 0 | 0 | 0 | 0 | 0 | 0 | 1 | 1 | 0 | 0 | 0 | 0 | 0 | 0 | 0 | 0 | 0 | 0 | 1 | 0 | 0 | 0 | 0 | 0 | 0 | 0 | 0 | 0 | 0 | 0 | 1 | 0 | 0 | 0 | 3 | 0 | 0 | 0 | 0 | 0 | 0 | 0 | 0 | 0 | 0 | 0 | 5 | 0 | 0 | 0 | 0 | 0 | 0 | 0 | 3 | 1 | 0 | 0 |
| 8 | 4 | 1 | 0 | 0 | 1 | 0 | 0 | 0 | 3 | 1 | 0 | 0 | 0 | 0 | 0 | 0 | 0 | 0 | 0 | 0 | 0 | 0 | 0 | 0 | 0 | 0 | 0 | 0 | 0 | 0 | 0 | 0 | 0 | 0 | 0 | 0 | 1 | 0 | 0 | 0 | 0 | 0 | 0 | 1 | 0 | 0 | 0 | 0 | 5 | 1 | 0 | 0 | 1 | 0 | 0 | 1 | 3 | 1 | 0 | 0 |
| 9 | 10 | 4 | 9 | 0 | 3 | 0 | 0 | 0 | 1 | 0 | 0 | 0 | 4 | 1 | 0 | 0 | 0 | 0 | 0 | 0 | 0 | 0 | 0 | 0 | 0 | 0 | 0 | 0 | 0 | 0 | 0 | 0 | 0 | 0 | 0 | 0 | 13 | 0 | 12 | 0 | 1 | 1 | 0 | 0 | 0 | 0 | 0 | 0 | 27 | 5 | 21 | 0 | 4 | 1 | 0 | 0 | 1 | 0 | 0 | 0 |
| 10 | 6 | 1 | 0 | 0 | 1 | 0 | 0 | 0 | 1 | 0 | 0 | 0 | 0 | 0 | 0 | 0 | 0 | 0 | 0 | 0 | 0 | 0 | 0 | 0 | 0 | 0 | 0 | 0 | 0 | 0 | 0 | 0 | 0 | 0 | 0 | 0 | 2 | 1 | 0 | 0 | 0 | 0 | 0 | 0 | 0 | 0 | 0 | 0 | 8 | 2 | 0 | 0 | 1 | 0 | 0 | 0 | 1 | 0 | 0 | 0 |

R = refusal to take test    B = shy bladder    A = adulterated    S = substituted

Data on Refusal Types for Four Test Types by FTA Region and Employer Size

| | Random | | | | | | Post-Accident | | | | | | Reasonable Suspicion | | | | | | Pre-Employment | | | | | | Total | | | | | |
|---|---|---|---|---|---|---|---|---|---|---|---|---|---|---|---|---|---|---|---|---|---|---|---|---|---|---|---|---|---|---|
| | Large | | Small | | Rural | | Large | | Small | | Rural | | Large | | Small | | Rural | | Large | | Small | | Rural | | Large | | Small | | Rural | |
| Region | RTT | SL | RTT | SL | RTT | SL | RTT | SL | RTT | SL | RTT | SL | RTT | SL | RTT | SL | RTT | SL | RTT | SL | RTT | SL | RTT | SL | RTT | SL | RTT | SL | RTT | SL |
| 1 | 0 | 1 | 0 | 0 | 0 | 0 | 1 | 0 | 0 | 0 | 0 | 0 | 0 | 0 | 0 | 0 | 0 | 0 | 0 | 0 | 0 | 0 | 0 | 0 | 1 | 0 | 0 | 0 | 0 | 0 |
| 2 | 0 | 0 | 0 | 0 | 0 | 0 | 2 | 1 | 0 | 0 | 0 | 0 | 0 | 0 | 0 | 0 | 0 | 0 | 0 | 0 | 0 | 0 | 0 | 0 | 4 | 1 | 0 | 0 | 0 | 0 |
| 3 | 2 | 0 | 0 | 0 | 0 | 0 | 0 | 0 | 0 | 0 | 0 | 0 | 0 | 0 | 0 | 0 | 0 | 0 | 0 | 1 | 0 | 0 | 0 | 0 | 0 | 1 | 0 | 0 | 0 | 0 |
| 4 | 0 | 0 | 0 | 0 | 1 | 0 | 1 | 0 | 0 | 0 | 0 | 0 | 0 | 0 | 0 | 0 | 0 | 0 | 0 | 0 | 0 | 0 | 0 | 0 | 1 | 0 | 0 | 0 | 1 | 0 |
| 5 | 0 | 0 | 0 | 0 | 0 | 0 | 5 | 1 | 0 | 0 | 0 | 0 | 0 | 0 | 0 | 0 | 0 | 0 | 0 | 0 | 0 | 0 | 0 | 0 | 6 | 3 | 0 | 0 | 0 | 0 |
| 6 | 1 | 2 | 0 | 0 | 0 | 0 | 1 | 0 | 0 | 0 | 0 | 0 | 2 | 0 | 0 | 0 | 1 | 0 | 0 | 0 | 0 | 0 | 0 | 0 | 3 | 0 | 0 | 0 | 1 | 0 |
| 7 | 0 | 0 | 0 | 0 | 2 | 1 | 0 | 0 | 0 | 0 | 0 | 0 | 0 | 0 | 0 | 0 | 0 | 0 | 0 | 0 | 0 | 0 | 0 | 0 | 0 | 0 | 0 | 0 | 2 | 1 |
| 8 | 0 | 0 | 0 | 0 | 0 | 0 | 0 | 0 | 0 | 0 | 0 | 0 | 0 | 0 | 0 | 0 | 0 | 0 | 0 | 0 | 0 | 0 | 0 | 0 | 0 | 0 | 0 | 0 | 0 | 0 |
| 9 | 0 | 0 | 0 | 0 | 0 | 0 | 1 | 0 | 0 | 0 | 0 | 0 | 2 | 0 | 0 | 0 | 0 | 0 | 0 | 0 | 0 | 0 | 0 | 0 | 4 | 0 | 0 | 0 | 0 | 0 |
| 10 | 1 | 0 | 0 | 0 | 1 | 0 | 0 | 0 | 0 | 0 | 0 | 1 | 0 | 0 | 0 | 0 | 0 | 0 | 0 | 0 | 0 | 0 | 0 | 0 | 0 | 0 | 0 | 0 | 1 | 1 |

RTT = refusal to take test          SL = shy lung

## 4.4 Data for Four Test Types by Type of Drug

The verified positive rates for each type of drug tested for are presented for each test type and for the four test types combined in the following graph. A table follows that provides the statistical basis for the rates. The table is followed by charts that show the percentage by drug type of the total drug type detections[9] for each test type and the four types combined. These rates and data are presented by employer type, employer size, and employee category later in this section.

Positive Rates by Test Type and Drug Type

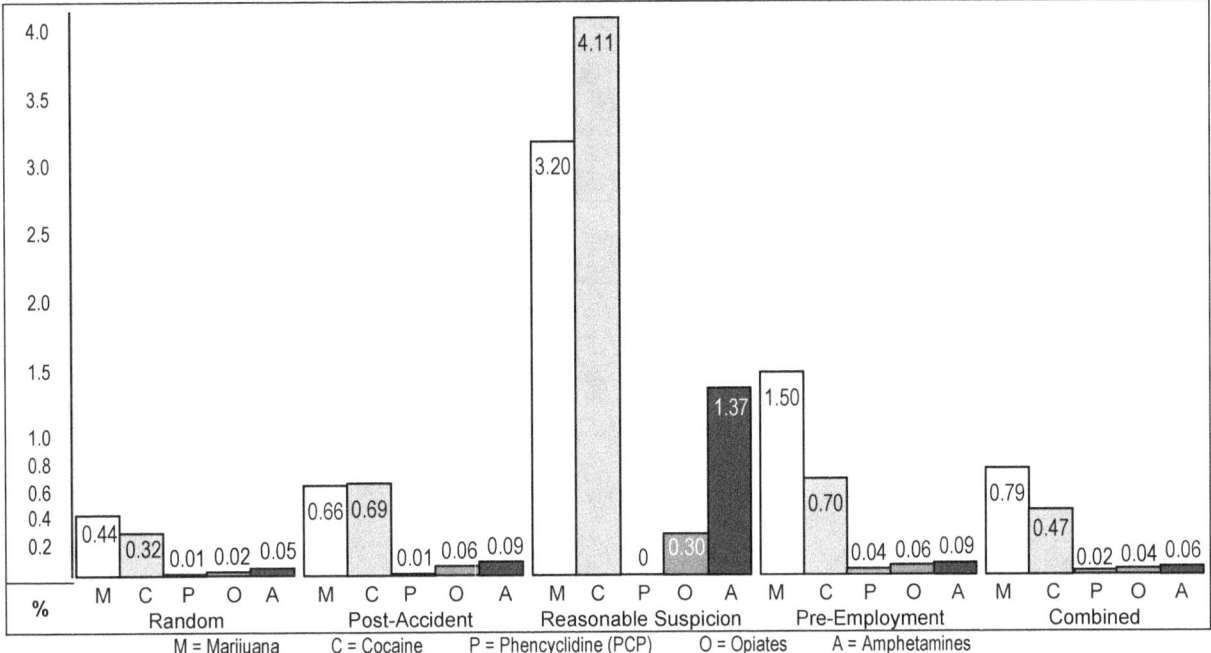

M = Marijuana     C = Cocaine     P = Phencyclidine (PCP)     O = Opiates     A = Amphetamines

---

[9] Because multiple drugs are sometimes detected in one specimen, the total number of drug detections may be greater than the total number of verified positives.

## Tests and Positives by Test Type and Drug Type

| | Testing Events | Verified Positives | | | | |
|---|---|---|---|---|---|---|
| | | Marijuana | Cocaine | PCP | Opiates | Amphetamines |
| Random | 135,297 | 599 | 433 | 10 | 27 | 61 |
| Post-Accident | 13,715 | 91 | 94 | 2 | 8 | 13 |
| Reasonable Suspicion | 657 | 21 | 27 | 0 | 2 | 9 |
| Pre-Employment | 65,774 | 984 | 463 | 28 | 40 | 56 |
| Total | 215,443 | 1,695 | 1,017 | 40 | 77 | 139 |

### Percentage by Drug Type of Total Drug Detections for Each Test Type

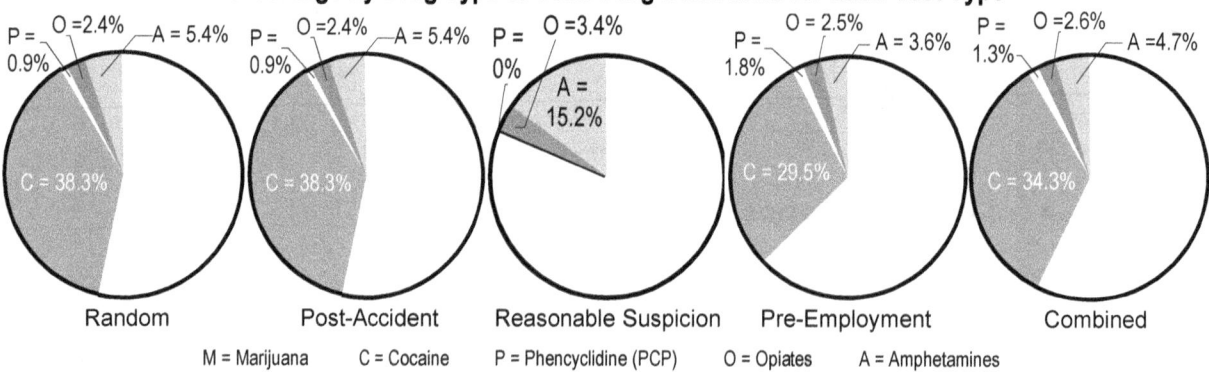

M = Marijuana   C = Cocaine   P = Phencyclidine (PCP)   O = Opiates   A = Amphetamines

### 4.4.1 Data for Four Test Types by Employer Type and Drug Type

The following graphs show the rates by drug type for each test type and the four test types combined by employer type. *The reasonable suspicion graph contains no columns for PCP because there were no PCP reasonable suspicion detections.*

### Positive Rates by Test Type, Employer Type, and Drug Type

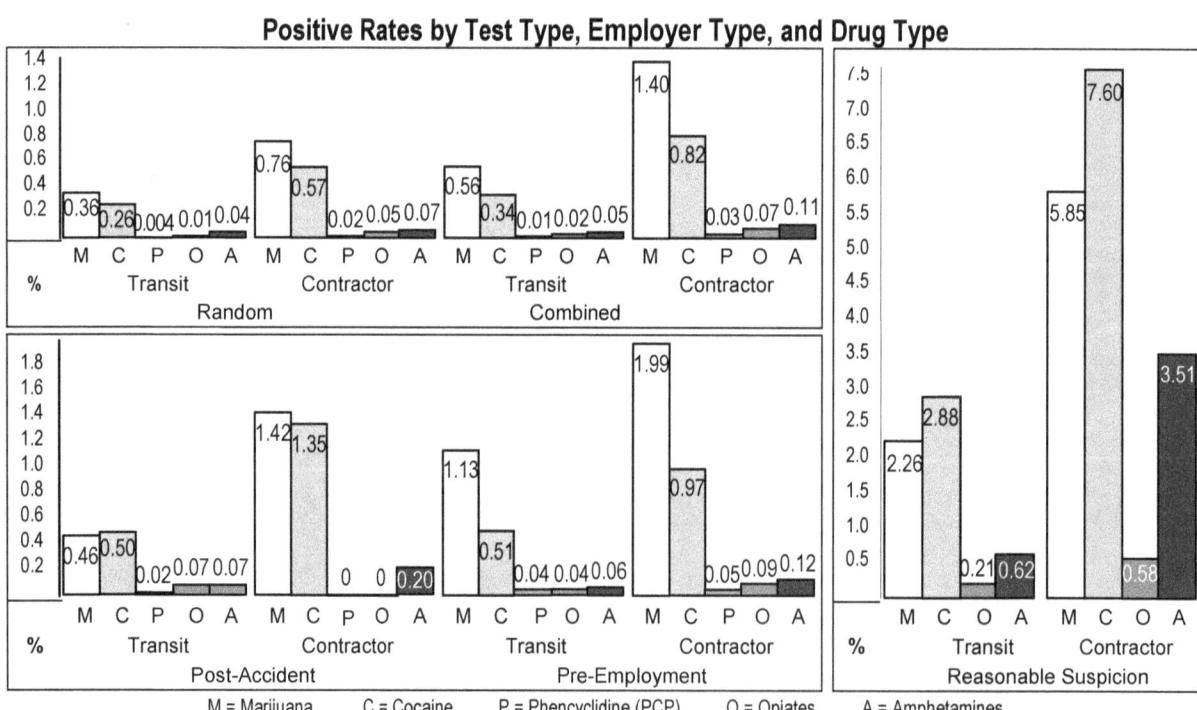

M = Marijuana   C = Cocaine   P = Phencyclidine (PCP)   O = Opiates   A = Amphetamines

The next table provides the statistical basis for the rates in the previous graphs. The table after that one shows the percentage by drug type of the total drug type detections for each test type and the four test types combined by employer type.

### Tests and Positives by Test Type, Employer Type, and Drug Type

| | Transit | | | | | | Contractor | | | | | |
|---|---|---|---|---|---|---|---|---|---|---|---|---|
| | TE | M | C | P | O | A | TE | M | C | P | O | A |
| Random | 108,239 | 394 | 280 | 5 | 13 | 43 | 27,058 | 205 | 153 | 5 | 14 | 18 |
| Post-Accident | 10,753 | 49 | 54 | 2 | 8 | 7 | 2,962 | 42 | 40 | 0 | 0 | 6 |
| Reasonable Suspicion | 486 | 11 | 14 | 0 | 1 | 3 | 171 | 10 | 13 | 0 | 1 | 6 |
| Pre-Employment | 37,597 | 423 | 191 | 15 | 14 | 23 | 28,177 | 561 | 272 | 13 | 26 | 33 |
| Total | 157,075 | 877 | 539 | 22 | 36 | 76 | 58,368 | 818 | 478 | 18 | 41 | 63 |

TE = testing events    M = Marijuana    C = Cocaine    P = Phencyclidine (PCP)    O = Opiates    A = Amphetamines

### Percentage by Drug Type of Total Drug Detections for Each Test Type by Employer Type

| | Transit | | | | | Contractor | | | | |
|---|---|---|---|---|---|---|---|---|---|---|
| | Marijuana | Cocaine | PCP | Opiates | Amphetamines | Marijuana | Cocaine | PCP | Opiates | Amphetamines |
| Random | 53.6 | 38.1 | 0.7 | 1.8 | 5.9 | 51.9 | 38.7 | 1.3 | 3.5 | 4.6 |
| Post-Accident | 40.8 | 45.0 | 1.7 | 6.7 | 5.8 | 47.7 | 45.5 | 0 | 0 | 6.8 |
| Reasonable Suspicion | 37.9 | 48.3 | 0 | 3.4 | 10.3 | 33.3 | 43.3 | 0 | 3.3 | 20.0 |
| Pre-Employment | 63.5 | 28.7 | 2.3 | 2.1 | 3.5 | 62.0 | 30.1 | 1.4 | 2.9 | 3.6 |
| Combined | 56.6 | 34.8 | 1.4 | 2.3 | 4.9 | 57.7 | 33.7 | 1.3 | 2.9 | 4.4 |

## 4.4.2 Data for Four Test Types by Employer Size and Drug Type

The next four graphs show the rates by drug type for each test type and for the four test types combined by employer size--the first graph for large employers

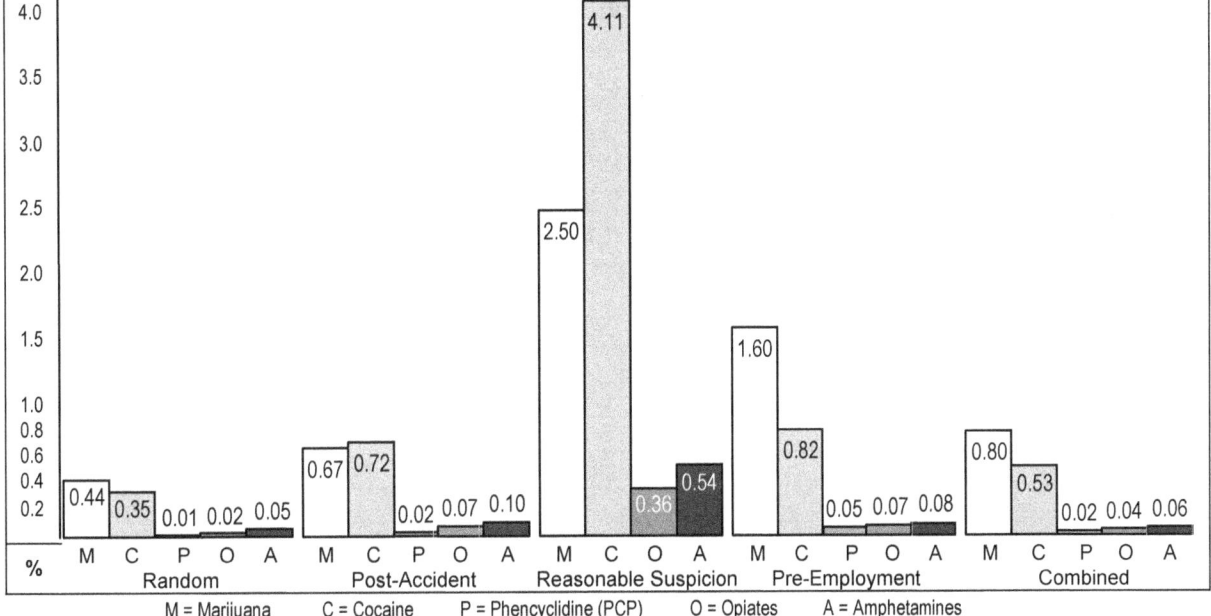

**Positive Rates by Test Type, Employer Size, and Drug Type—Large Employers**

M = Marijuana    C = Cocaine    P = Phencyclidine (PCP)    O = Opiates    A = Amphetamines

and the other three for small and rural employers. *The reasonable suspicion graphs contain no columns for PCP because there were no PCP reasonable suspicion detections.* Two tables follow the graphs. The first provides the statistical basis for the rates. The second shows the percentage by drug type of the total drug type detections for each test type by employer size.

### Positive Rates by Test Type, Employer Size, and Drug Type—Small and Rural

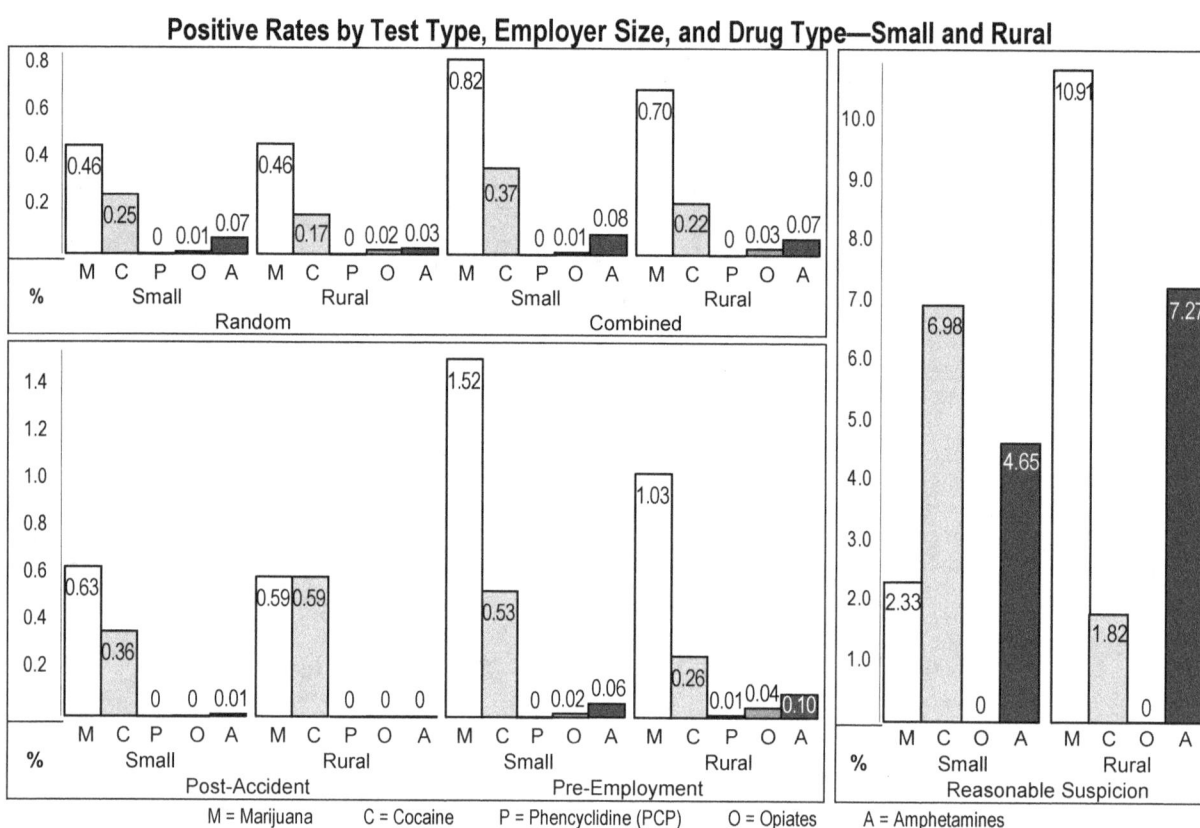

M = Marijuana    C = Cocaine    P = Phencyclidine (PCP)    O = Opiates    A = Amphetamines

### Tests and Positives by Test Type, Employer Size, and Drug Type

| | Large | | | | | Small | | | | | Rural | | | | |
|---|---|---|---|---|---|---|---|---|---|---|---|---|---|---|---|
| | TE | M | C | P | O | A | TE | M | C | P | O | A | TE | M | C | P | O | A |
| Random | 108,735 | 477 | 382 | 10 | 23 | 49 | 8,556 | 39 | 21 | 0 | 1 | 6 | 18,006 | 83 | 30 | 0 | 3 | 6 |
| Post-Accident | 11,592 | 78 | 84 | 2 | 8 | 12 | 1,104 | 7 | 4 | 0 | 0 | 1 | 1,019 | 6 | 6 | 0 | 0 | 0 |
| Reasonable Suspicion | 559 | 14 | 23 | 0 | 2 | 3 | 43 | 1 | 3 | 0 | 0 | 2 | 55 | 6 | 1 | 0 | 0 | 4 |
| Pre-Employment | 49,860 | 797 | 409 | 27 | 34 | 42 | 4,678 | 71 | 25 | 0 | 1 | 3 | 11,236 | 116 | 29 | 1 | 5 | 11 |
| Total | 170,746 | 1,366 | 898 | 39 | 67 | 106 | 14,381 | 118 | 53 | 0 | 2 | 12 | 30,316 | 211 | 66 | 1 | 8 | 21 |

TE = testing events    M = Marijuana    C = Cocaine    P = Phencyclidine (PCP)    O = Opiates    A = Amphetamines

### Percentage by Drug Type of Total Drug Detections for Each Test Type by Employer Size

| | Large | | | | | Small | | | | | Rural | | | | |
|---|---|---|---|---|---|---|---|---|---|---|---|---|---|---|---|
| | M | C | P | O | A | M | C | P | O | A | M | C | P | O | A |
| Random | 50.7 | 40.6 | 1.1 | 2.4 | 5.2 | 58.2 | 31.3 | 0 | 1.5 | 9.0 | 68.0 | 24.6 | 0 | 2.5 | 4.9 |
| Post-Accident | 42.4 | 45.7 | 1.1 | 4.3 | 6.5 | 58.3 | 33.3 | 0 | 0 | 8.3 | 50.0 | 50.0 | 0 | 0 | 0 |
| Reasonable Suspicion | 33.3 | 54.8 | 0 | 4.8 | 7.1 | 16.7 | 50.0 | 0 | 0 | 33.3 | 54.5 | 9.1 | 0 | 0 | 36.4 |
| Pre-Employment | 60.9 | 31.2 | 2.1 | 2.6 | 3.2 | 71.0 | 25.0 | 0 | 1.0 | 3.0 | 71.6 | 17.9 | 0.6 | 3.1 | 6.8 |
| Combined | 55.2 | 36.3 | 1.6 | 2.7 | 4.3 | 63.8 | 28.6 | 0 | 1.1 | 6.5 | 68.7 | 21.5 | 0.3 | 2.6 | 6.8 |

M = Marijuana    C = Cocaine    P = Phencyclidine (PCP)    O = Opiates    A = Amphetamines

## 4.4.3 Data for Four Test Types by Employee Category and Drug Type

The following five graphs show the rates by drug type for each test type and for the four test types combined by employee category. A graph is presented for the four test types combined and for each test type. Two tables follow the graphs. The first provides the statistical basis for the rates. The second shows the percentage by drug type of the total drug type detections for each test type and the four test types combined by employee category.

**Positive Rates for Four Test Types Combined by Employee Category and Drug Type**

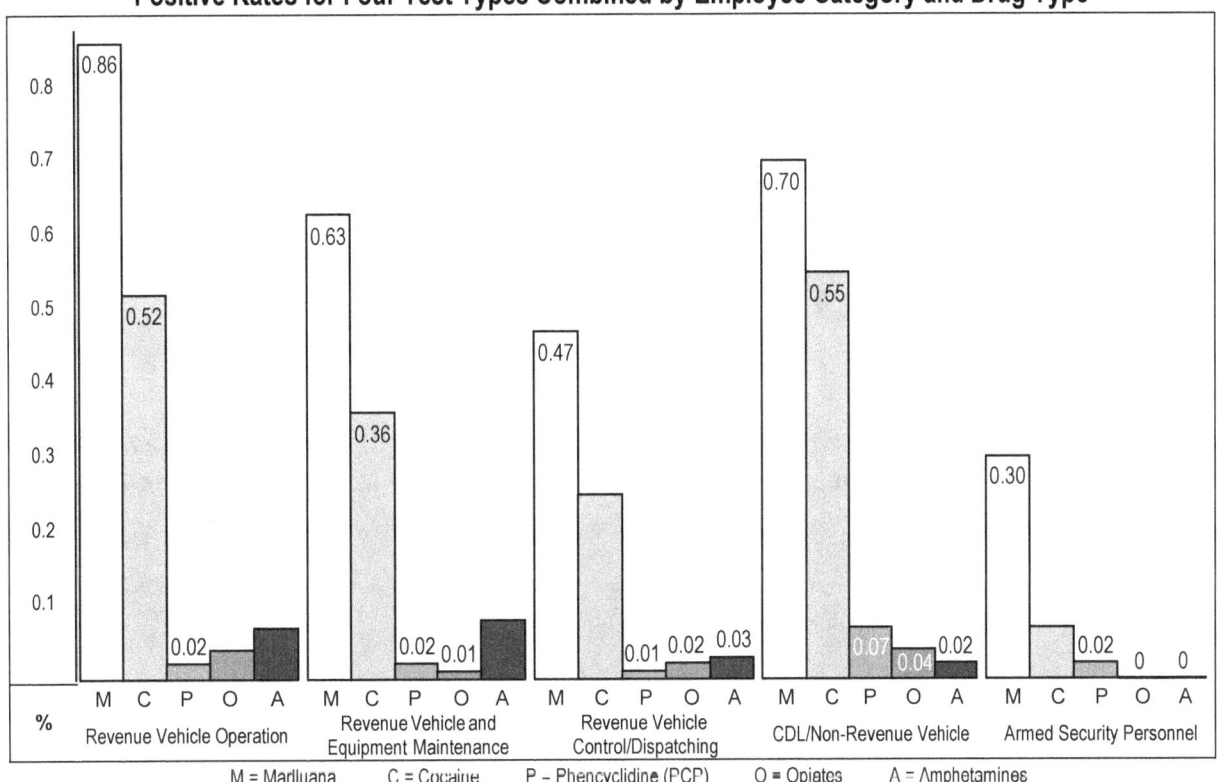

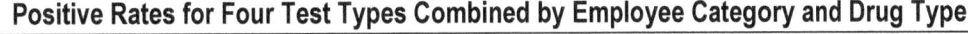

**Random Positive Rates by Employee Category and Drug Type**

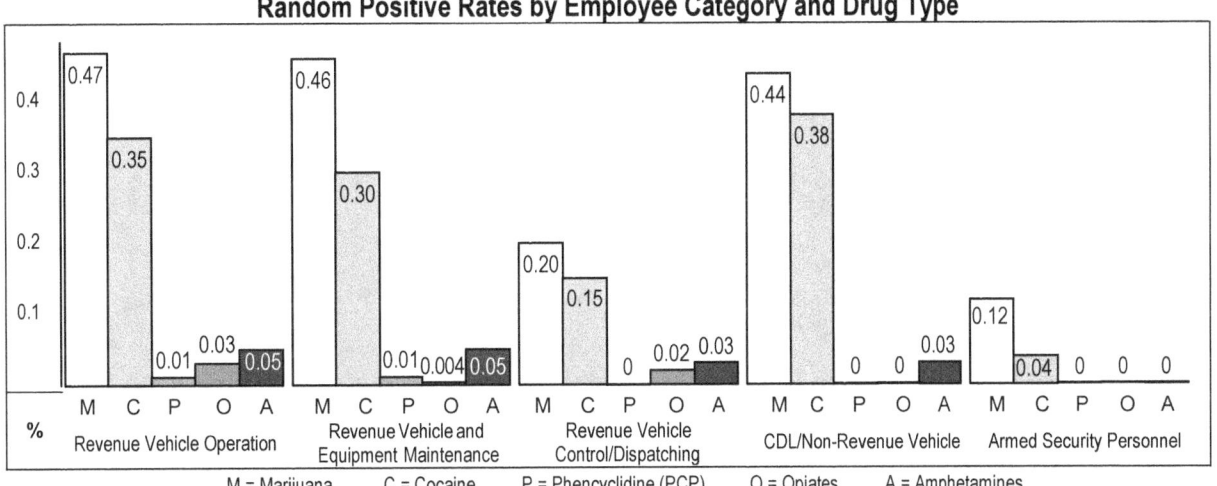

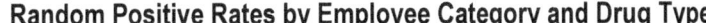

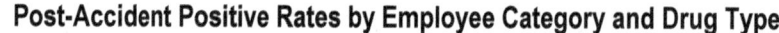

**Post-Accident Positive Rates by Employee Category and Drug Type**

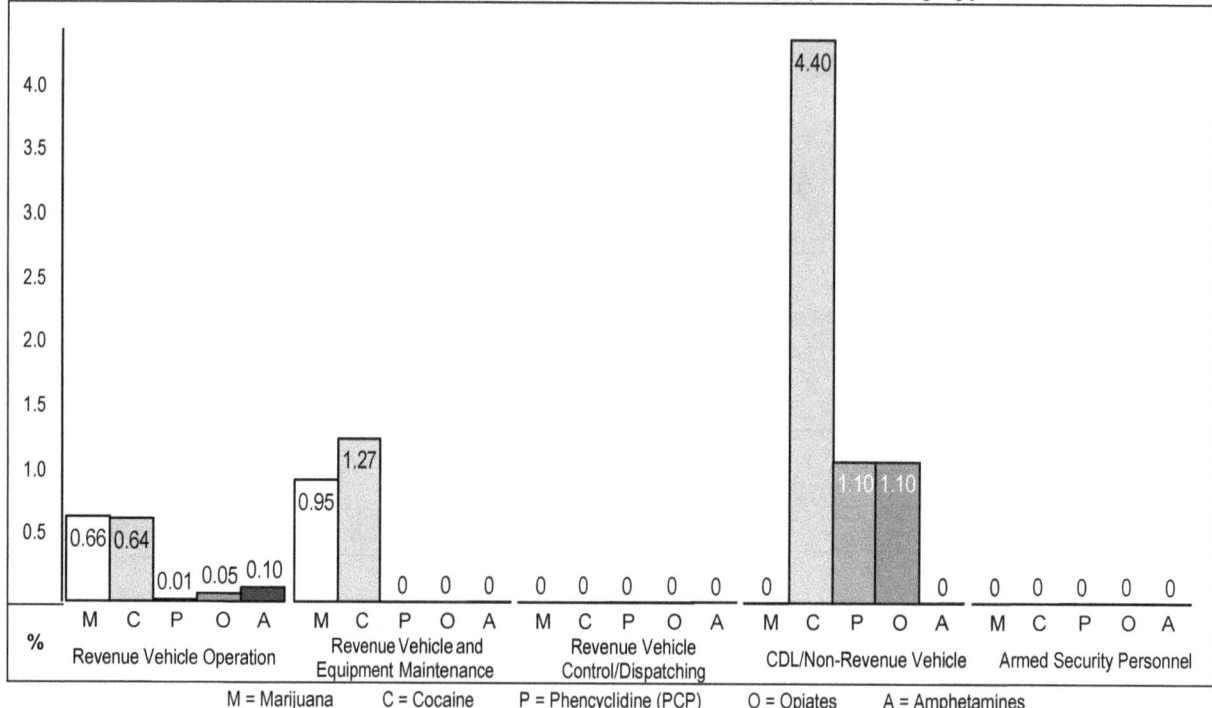

Note: *The following graph does not contain columns for PCP because there were no PCP detections in any reasonable suspicion tests—i.e., "0" in the reasonable suspicion column of the graph on page 4-29.*

**Reasonable Suspicion Positive Rates by Employee Category and Drug Type**

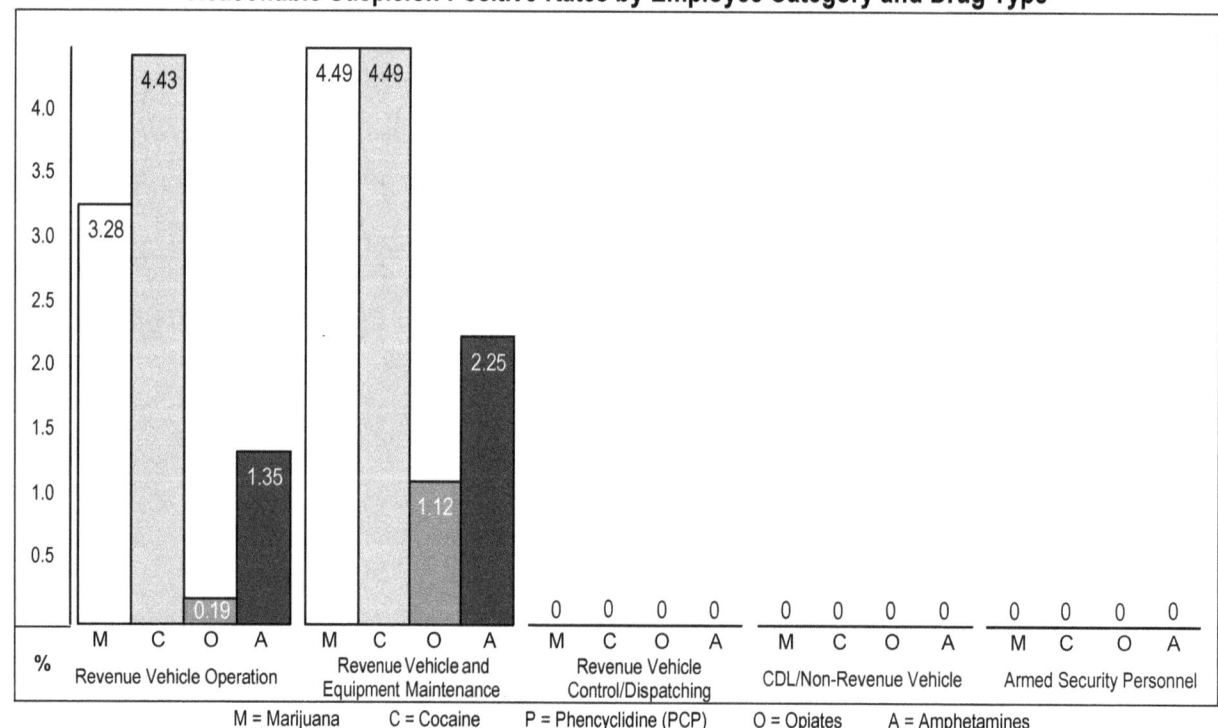

## Pre-Employment Positive Rates by Employee Category and Drug Type

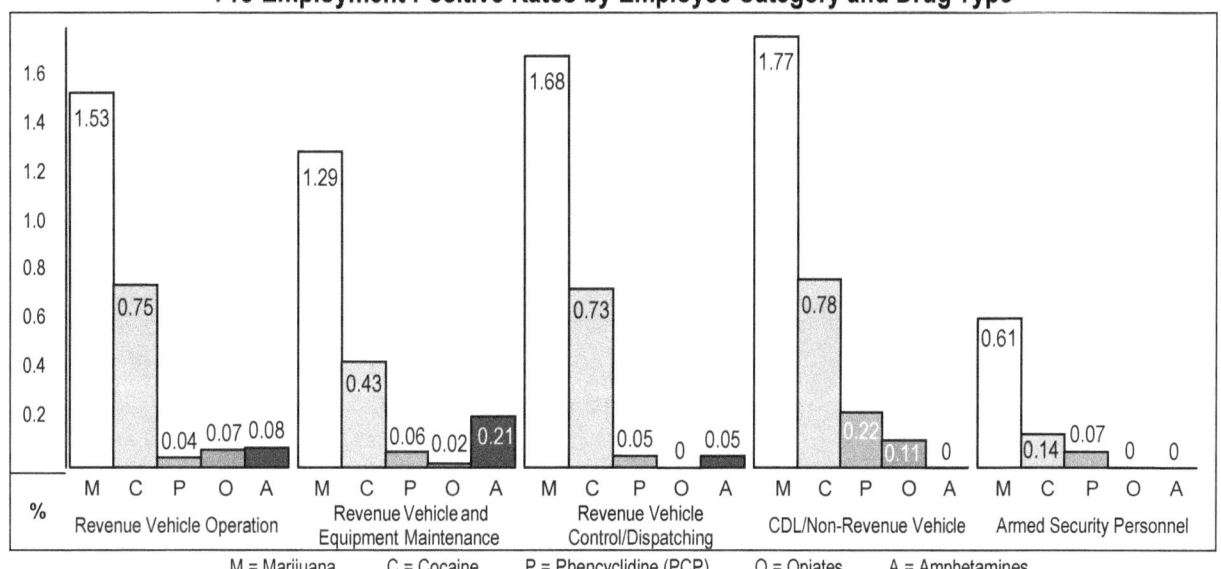

M = Marijuana    C = Cocaine    P = Phencyclidine (PCP)    O = Opiates    A = Amphetamines

## Tests and Positives, and Refusals by Test Type, Employee Category, and Drug Type

| | | Testing Events | Verified Positives | | | | |
|---|---|---|---|---|---|---|---|
| | | | Marijuana | Cocaine | PCP | Opiates | Amphetamines |
| Random | RVO | 92,496 | 436 | 322 | 8 | 24 | 43 |
| | RV&EM | 27,602 | 127 | 84 | 2 | 1 | 14 |
| | RVC/D | 9,515 | 19 | 14 | 0 | 2 | 3 |
| | CDL/N-RV | 3,189 | 14 | 12 | 0 | 0 | 1 |
| | ASP | 2,495 | 3 | 1 | 0 | 0 | 0 |
| Post-Accident | RVO | 12,783 | 85 | 82 | 1 | 7 | 13 |
| | RV&EM | 630 | 6 | 8 | 0 | 0 | 0 |
| | RVC/D | 107 | 0 | 0 | 0 | 0 | 0 |
| | CDL/N-RV | 91 | 0 | 4 | 1 | 1 | 0 |
| | ASP | 104 | 0 | 0 | 0 | 0 | 0 |
| Reasonable Suspicion | RVO | 519 | 17 | 23 | 0 | 1 | 7 |
| | RV&EM | 89 | 4 | 4 | 0 | 1 | 2 |
| | RVC/D | 28 | 0 | 0 | 0 | 0 | 0 |
| | CDL/N-RV | 20 | 0 | 0 | 0 | 0 | 0 |
| | ASP | 1 | 0 | 0 | 0 | 0 | 0 |
| Pre-Employment | RVO | 54,936 | 841 | 411 | 20 | 38 | 42 |
| | RV&EM | 6,271 | 81 | 27 | 4 | 1 | 13 |
| | RVC/D | 2,197 | 37 | 16 | 1 | 0 | 1 |
| | CDL/N-RV | 903 | 16 | 7 | 2 | 1 | 0 |
| | ASP | 1,467 | 9 | 2 | 1 | 0 | 0 |
| Total | RVO | 160,734 | 1,379 | 838 | 29 | 70 | 105 |
| | RV&EM | 34,592 | 218 | 123 | 6 | 3 | 29 |
| | RVC/D | 11,847 | 56 | 30 | 1 | 2 | 4 |
| | CDL/N-RV | 4,203 | 1,653 | 991 | 36 | 75 | 138 |
| | ASP | 4,067 | 12 | 3 | 1 | 0 | 0 |

RVO = Revenue Vehicle Operation          RV&EM = Revenue Vehicle and Equipment Maintenance

RVC/D = Revenue Vehicle Control/Dispatching          CDL/N-RV = CDL/Non-Revenue Vehicle          ASP = Armed Security Personnel

**Percentage by Drug Type of Total Drug Detections for Each Test Type by Employee Category**

| | Revenue Vehicle Operation | | | | | Revenue Vehicle and Equipment Maintenance | | | | | Revenue Vehicle Control/Dispatching | | | | | CDL/Non-Revenue Vehicle | | | | | Armed Security Personnel | | | | |
|---|---|---|---|---|---|---|---|---|---|---|---|---|---|---|---|---|---|---|---|---|---|---|---|---|---|
| | M | C | P | O | A | M | C | P | O | A | M | C | P | O | A | M | C | P | O | A | M | C | P | O | A |
| Random | 52.3 | 38.7 | 1.0 | 2.9 | 5.2 | 55.7 | 36.9 | 0.9 | 0.4 | 6.1 | 50.0 | 36.8 | 0 | 5.3 | 7.9 | 51.9 | 44.4 | 0 | 0 | 3.7 | 75.0 | 25.0 | 0 | 0 | 0 |
| Post-Accident | 45.2 | 43.6 | 0.5 | 3.7 | 6.9 | 42.9 | 57.1 | 0 | 0 | 0 | 0 | 0 | 0 | 0 | 0 | 66.7 | 16.7 | 16.7 | 0 | 0 | 0 | 0 | 0 | 0 | 0 |
| Reasonable Suspicion | 35.4 | 47.9 | 0 | 2.1 | 14.6 | 36.4 | 36.4 | 0 | 9.1 | 18.2 | 0 | 0 | 0 | 0 | 0 | 0 | 0 | 0 | 0 | 0 | 0 | 0 | 0 | 0 | 0 |
| Pre-Employment | 62.2 | 30.4 | 1.5 | 2.8 | 3.1 | 64.3 | 21.4 | 3.2 | 0.8 | 10.3 | 67.3 | 29.1 | 1.8 | 0 | 1.8 | 61.5 | 26.9 | 7.7 | 3.9 | 0 | 75.0 | 16.7 | 8.3 | 0 | 0 |
| Combined | 57.0 | 34.6 | 1.2 | 2.9 | 4.3 | 57.5 | 32.5 | 1.6 | 0.8 | 7.7 | 60.2 | 32.3 | 1.1 | 2.1 | 4.3 | 50.8 | 39.0 | 5.1 | 3.4 | 1.7 | 75.0 | 18.8 | 6.3 | 0.0 | 0.0 |

M = Marijuana    C = Cocaine    P = Phencyclidine (PCP)    O = Opiates    A = Amphetamines

## 4.5 Confirmed Alcohol Specimens Between 0.02 and 0.039

The table at right presents the number of confirmed alcohol specimens with levels between 0.02 and 0.039 by test type, the percentage of such specimens of the total number of testing events (events), and the total number of testing events. Those numbers are subdivided by employer type, employer size, employer size and type combined, employee category, and FTA region, respectively, in the tables that follow. (For all test types except reasonable suspicion and for all the types combined, the percentages of the entire number of tests and the percentage of the total number with levels lower than 0.04 are the same after rounding. Both rates are included in the "percent of tests" column for reasonable suspicion tests where the rates differ.)

**Alcohol Confirmations Between 0.02 and 0.039 by Test Type**

| | Percent of Events | 0.02 to 0.039 | Testing Events |
|---|---|---|---|
| Random | 0.04 | 18 | 42,317 |
| Post-Accident | 0.04 | 5 | 12,490 |
| Reasonable Suspicion | 4.68/ 5.25* | 29 | 620 |
| Pre-Employment | 0.01 | 1 | 9,672 |
| Total | 0.08 | 53 | 65,099 |

**Alcohol Confirmations Between 0.02 and 0.039 by Test Type and Employer Type**

| | Transit | | | Contractor | | |
|---|---|---|---|---|---|---|
| | Percent of Events | 0.02 to 0.039 | Testing Events | Percent of Events | 0.02 to 0.039 | Testing Events |
| Random | 0.04 | 15 | 34,446 | 0.04 | 3 | 7,871 |
| Post-Accident | 0.04 | 4 | 10,038 | 0.04 | 1 | 2,452 |
| Reasonable Suspicion | 4.33/ 4.78* | 20 | 462 | 5.70/ 6.72* | 9 | 158 |
| Pre-Employment | 0 | 0 | 6, 650 | 0.03 | 1 | 3,022 |
| Total | 0.08 | 39 | 51,596 | 0.10 | 14 | 13,503 |

*Bottom number is the percentage of the number of tests minus confirmed positives. Both percentages are the same for the other reasonable suspicion breakdowns and for the other test types.

**Alcohol Confirmations Between 0.02 and 0.039 by Test Type and Employer Size**

| | Large | | | Small | | | Rural | | |
|---|---|---|---|---|---|---|---|---|---|
| | Percent of Events | 0.02 to 0.039 | Testing Events | Percent of Events | 0.02 to 0.039 | Tests | Percent of Events | 0.02 to 0.039 | Testing Events |
| Random | 0.04 | 14 | 108,735 | 0 | 0 | 8,556 | 0.08 | 4 | 18,006 |
| Post-Accident | 0.03 | 3 | 11,592 | 0.22 | 2 | 1,104 | 0 | 0 | 1,019 |
| Reasonable Suspicion | 4.28/ 4.77* | 23 | 559 | 5.00/ 5.88* | 2 | 43 | 9.52/ 11.11* | 4 | 55 |
| Pre-Employment | 0.01 | 1 | 49,860 | 0 | 0 | 4,678 | 0 | 0 | 11,236 |
| Total | 0.08 | 41 | 170,746 | 0.10 | 4 | 14,381 | 0.12 | 8 | 30,316 |

*The bottom number is the percentage of the number of tests minus confirmed positives. Both percentages are the same for the other reasonable suspicion breakdowns and for the other test types.

## Alcohol Confirmations Between 0.02 and 0.039 by Test Type, Employer Size, and Employer Type

| | Large Transit % of Events | Large Transit .02-.039 | Large Transit Testing Events | Large Contractor % of Events | Large Contractor .02-.039 | Large Contractor Testing Events | Small Transit % of Events | Small Transit .02-.039 | Small Transit Testing Events | Small Contractor % of Events | Small Contractor .02-.039 | Small Contractor Testing Events | Rural Transit % of Events | Rural Transit .02-.039 | Rural Transit Testing Events | Rural Contractor % of Events | Rural Contractor .02-.039 | Rural Contractor Testing Events |
|---|---|---|---|---|---|---|---|---|---|---|---|---|---|---|---|---|---|---|
| Random | 0.04 | 11 | 27,875 | 0.04 | 3 | 6,824 | 0 | 0 | 1,974 | 0 | 0 | 556 | 0.09 | 4 | 4,597 | 0 | 0 | 491 |
| Post-Accident | 0.02 | 2 | 8,578 | 0.04 | 1 | 2,275 | 0.26 | 2 | 780 | 0 | 0 | 119 | 0 | 0 | 680 | 0 | 0 | 58 |
| Reasonable Suspicion | 4.23/4.62* | 17 | 402 | 4.41/5.26* | 6 | 136 | 0 | 0 | 25 | 13.30/15.38* | 2 | 15 | 8.57/10.34* | 3 | 35 | 14.29 | 1 | 7 |
| Pre-Employment | 0 | 0 | 5,439 | 0.04 | 1 | 2,851 | 0 | 0 | 362 | 0 | 0 | 94 | 0 | 0 | 849 | 0 | 0 | 77 |
| Total | 0.07 | 30 | 42,294 | 0.09 | 1 | 12,086 | 0.06 | 2 | 3,141 | 0.26 | 7 | 784 | 0.11 | 7 | 6,161 | 0.16 | 5 | 633 |

*The bottom number is the percentage of the number of tests minus confirmed positives. Both percentages are the same for the other reasonable suspicion breakdowns and for the other test types.

## Alcohol Confirmations Between 0.02 and 0.039 by Test Type and Employee Category

| | Revenue Vehicle Operation % of Events | Revenue Vehicle Operation .02-.039 | Revenue Vehicle Operation Testing Events | Revenue Vehicle and Equipment Maintenance % of Events | Revenue Vehicle and Equipment Maintenance .02-.039 | Revenue Vehicle and Equipment Maintenance Testing Events | Revenue Vehicle Control/Dispatching % of Events | Revenue Vehicle Control/Dispatching .02-.039 | Revenue Vehicle Control/Dispatching Testing Events | CDL/Non-Revenue Vehicle % of Events | CDL/Non-Revenue Vehicle .02-.039 | CDL/Non-Revenue Vehicle Testing Events | Armed Security Personnel % of Events | Armed Security Personnel .02-.039 | Armed Security Personnel Testing Events |
|---|---|---|---|---|---|---|---|---|---|---|---|---|---|---|---|
| Random | 0.05 | 15 | 28,702 | 0.03 | 3 | 8,587 | 0 | 0 | 2,882 | 0 | 0 | 1,254 | 0 | 0 | 892 |
| Post-Accident | 0.04 | 5 | 11,719 | 0 | 0 | 539 | 0 | 0 | 89 | 0 | 0 | 79 | 0 | 0 | 64 |
| Reasonable Suspicion | 3.87/4.37* | 19 | 491 | 8.54/9.33* | 7 | 82 | 6.06/6.25* | 2 | 33 | 7.14/10.00* | 1 | 14 | 0 | 0 | 0 |
| Pre-Employment | 0.01 | 1 | 7,671 | 0 | 0 | 1,120 | 0 | 0 | 285 | 0 | 0 | 154 | 0 | 0 | 442 |
| Total | 0.08 | 40 | 48,583 | 0.10 | 10 | 10,328 | 0.06 | 2 | 3,289 | 0.07 | 1 | 1,501 | 0 | 0 | 1,398 |

*The bottom number is the percentage of the number of tests minus confirmed positives. Both percentages are the same for the other reasonable suspicion breakdowns and for the other test types.

## Alcohol Confirmations Between 0.02 and 0.039 for Four Test Types by FTA Region

| Region | Random Percent of Events | Random 0.02 to 0.039 | Random Testing Events | Post-Accident Percent of Events | Post-Accident 0.02 to 0.039 | Post-Accident Testing Events | Reasonable Suspicion Percent of Events | Reasonable Suspicion 0.02 to 0.039 | Reasonable Suspicion Testing Events | Pre-Employment Percent of Events | Pre-Employment 0.02 to 0.039 | Pre-Employment Testing Events | Total Percent of Events | Total 0.02 to 0.039 | Total Testing Events |
|---|---|---|---|---|---|---|---|---|---|---|---|---|---|---|---|
| 1 | 0.22 | 2 | 1,342 | 0 | 0 | 435 | 15.38 | 2 | 13 | 0 | 0 | 255 | 0.20 | 4 | 2,006 |
| 2 | 0.02 | 2 | 9,182 | 0.05 | 1 | 1,930 | 3.86 | 8 | 207 | 0 | 0 | 2,010 | 0.08 | 11 | 13,239 |
| 3 | 0.02 | 1 | 5,962 | 0 | 0 | 1,153 | 2.33 | 2 | 86 | 0 | 0 | 2,428 | 0.03 | 3 | 9,498 |
| 4 | 0.04 | 2 | 5,332 | 0 | 0 | 2,501 | 5.13 | 2 | 39 | 0 | 0 | 1,274 | 0.05 | 4 | 8,868 |
| 5 | 0.04 | 2 | 5,711 | 0 | 0 | 2,489 | 2.83 | 3 | 106 | 0 | 0 | 691 | 0.06 | 5 | 8,870 |
| 6 | 0.02 | 1 | 4,870 | 0.27 | 3 | 1,296 | 0 | 0 | 25 | 0 | 0 | 1,021 | 0.06 | 4 | 7,019 |
| 7 | 0.18 | 2 | 1,118 | 0.33 | 1 | 351 | 0 | 0 | 12 | 0 | 0 | 22 | 0.21 | 3 | 1,451 |
| 8 | 0.09 | 1 | 1,061 | 0 | 0 | 338 | 29.17 | 7 | 24 | 0 | 0 | 84 | 0.55 | 8 | 1,445 |
| 9 | 0.08 | 4 | 5,186 | 0 | 0 | 2,693 | 5.00 | 4 | 80 | 0.06 | 1 | 1,811 | 0.09 | 9 | 9,547 |
| 10 | 0.04 | 1 | 2,553 | 0 | 0 | 529 | 3.57 | 1 | 28 | 0 | 0 | 76 | 0.06 | 2 | 3,156 |

*The bottom number is the percentage of the number of tests minus confirmed positives. Both percentages are the same for the other reasonable suspicion breakdowns and for the other test types.

# 5. Drug and Alcohol Data for Return to Duty Testing and Follow-up Testing

This chapter presents test data on persons who have been returned to FTA safety-sensitive duty after testing positive for drugs or alcohol or refusing to submit to a required test and who have subsequently completed a rehabilitation program designed by a substance abuse professional (SAP).  Section 5.1 summarizes data for return to duty tests performed in 2003.  Section 5.2 summarizes data for follow-up tests performed in 2003.  The results are sorted and presented by employer type, employer size, employee category, FTA region, and drug type.

## 5.1 Return to Duty Test Data

The combined percentage of positive tests plus test refusals for return to duty drug tests and alcohol tests[10] are shown in the graph at right.  The statistical basis for those rates is provided in the table next to the graph.  The rates are subdivided by employer type and size, by employee category, by

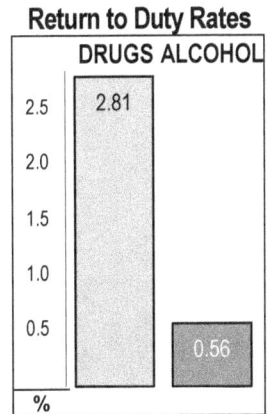

**Return to Duty Rates**

| Return to Duty Tests, Positives, and Refusals | Drugs | Alcohol |
|---|---|---|
| Testing Events | 1,283 | 713 |
| Refusals + Positives | 36 | 4 |
| Positives | 28 | 3 |
| Total Refusals | 8 | 1 |
| Refusal to take test | 5 | 1 |
| Shy Bladder/Lung | 2 | 0 |
| Adulterated | 0 | N. A. |
| Substituted | 1 | N. A. |
| Refusal Rate | 0.624 | 0.140 |

FTA region, and by type of drug later in this section.

### 5.1.1 Return to Duty Test Data by Employer Type and Size

The rates in the preceding graph are subdivided by employer type, by employer size, and by employer size and type, respectively, in the three graphs on the next page.  The three tables that follow the graphs provide the statistical basis for the rates.

> *The graph (at right on the next page) showing employer size rates subdivided by employer type shows alcohol rates for only large transit employers because no confirmed alcohol positives or test refusals were reported by small or rural employers or by contractors.*

---

[10] A positive alcohol test is a confirmed specimen with a breath alcohol level of at least 0.04.

*2003 Annual Report*

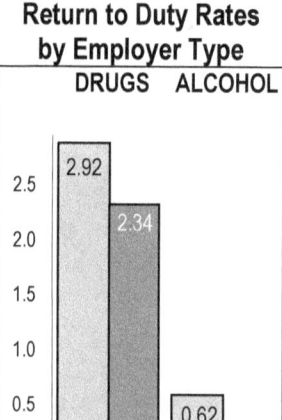

**Return to Duty Rates by Employer Type**

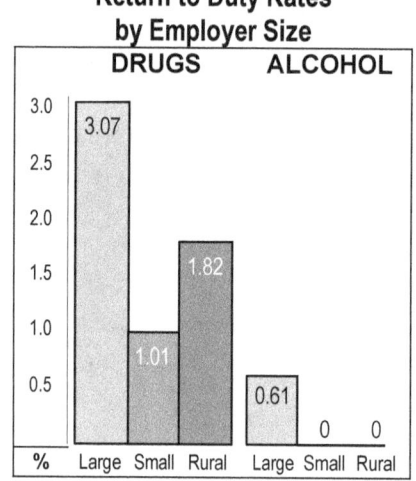

**Return to Duty Rates by Employer Size**

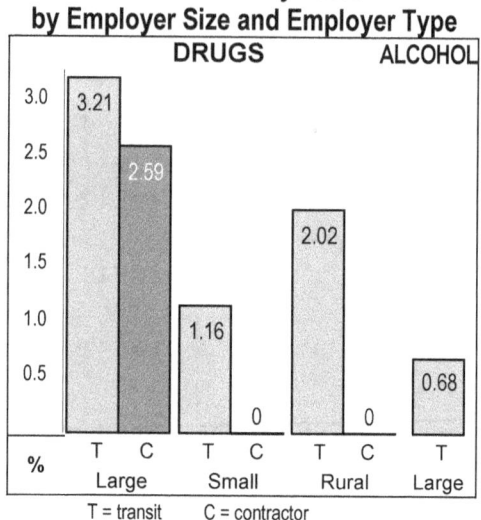

**Return to Duty Rates by Employer Size and Employer Type**

### Return to Duty Tests, Positives, and Refusals by Employer Type

|  | Drugs | | Alcohol | |
|---|---|---|---|---|
|  | Transit | Contractor | Transit | Contractor |
| Testing Events | 1,027 | 256 | 642 | 71 |
| Refusals + Positives | 30 | 6 | 4 | 0 |
| Positives | 24 | 4 | 3 | 0 |
| Total Refusals | 6 | 2 | 1 | 0 |
| Refusal to take test | 4 | 1 | 1 | 0 |
| Shy Bladder/Lung | 1 | 1 | 0 | 0 |
| Adulterated | 0 | 0 | N. A. | N. A. |
| Substituted | 1 | 0 | N. A. | N. A. |
| Refusal Rate | 0.584 | 0.781 | 0.156 | 0 |

### Return to Duty Tests, Positives, and Refusals by Employer Size

|  | Drugs | | | Alcohol | | |
|---|---|---|---|---|---|---|
|  | Large | Small | Rural | Large | Small | Rural |
| Testing Events | 1,074 | 99 | 110 | 658 | 34 | 21 |
| R + P | 33 | 1 | 2 | 4 | 0 | 0 |
| Positives (P) | 26 | 1 | 1 | 3 | 0 | 0 |
| Total Refusals (R) | 7 | 0 | 1 | 1 | 0 | 0 |
| Refusal to take test | 5 | 0 | 0 | 1 | 0 | 0 |
| Shy Bladder/Lung | 1 | 0 | 1 | 0 | 0 | 0 |
| Adulterated | 0 | 0 | 0 | N. A. | N. A. | N. A. |
| Substituted | 1 | 0 | 0 | N. A. | N. A. | N. A. |
| Refusal Rate | 0.652 | 0.000 | 0.909 | 0.152 | 0 | 0 |

### Return to Duty Tests, Positives, and Refusals by Employer Size and Employer Type

|  | Drugs | | | | | | Alcohol | | | | | |
|---|---|---|---|---|---|---|---|---|---|---|---|---|
|  | Large | | Small | | Rural | | Large | | Small | | Rural | |
|  | Transit | Contractor | Transit | Contractor | Transit | Contractor | Transit | Contractor | Transit | Contractor | Transit | Contractor |
| Testing Events | 842 | 232 | 86 | 13 | 99 | 11 | 592 | 66 | 30 | 4 | 20 | 1 |
| Refusals + Positives | 27 | 6 | 1 | 0 | 2 | 0 | 4 | 0 | 0 | 0 | 0 | 0 |
| Positives | 22 | 4 | 1 | 0 | 1 | 0 | 3 | 0 | 0 | 0 | 0 | 0 |
| Total Refusals | 5 | 2 | 0 | 0 | 1 | 0 | 1 | 0 | 0 | 0 | 0 | 0 |
| Refusal to take test | 4 | 1 | 0 | 0 | 0 | 0 | 1 | 0 | 0 | 0 | 0 | 0 |
| Shy Bladder/Lung | 0 | 1 | 0 | 0 | 1 | 0 | 0 | 0 | 0 | 0 | 0 | 0 |
| Adulterated | 0 | 0 | 0 | 0 | 0 | 0 | N. A. | N. A. | N. A. | N. A. | N. A. | N. A. |
| Substituted | 1 | 0 | 0 | 0 | 0 | 0 | N. A. | N. A. | N. A. | N. A. | N. A. | N. A. |
| Refusal Rate | 0.594 | 0.862 | 0.000 | 0.000 | 1.010 | 0.000 | 0.169 | 0 | 0 | 0 | 0 | 0 |

## 5.1.2  Return to Duty Test Data by Employee Category

The following graph shows the rates for return to duty drug tests and alcohol tests by employee category. The table next to it provides the statistical basis for the rates.

## Return to Duty Rates by Employee Category

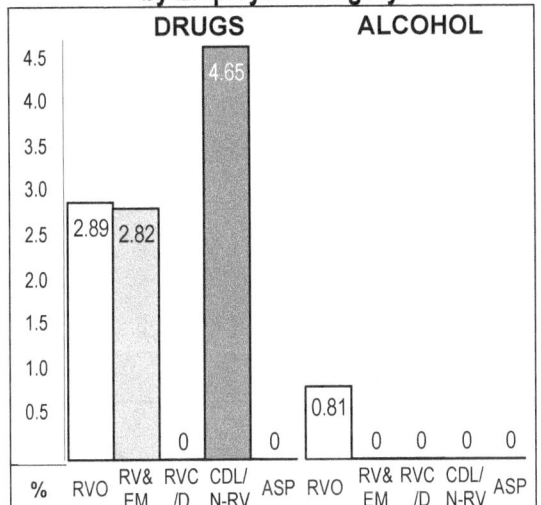

DRUGS      ALCOHOL

RVO = Revenue Vehicle Operation
RV&EM = Revenue Vehicle and Equipment Maintenance
RVC/D = Revenue Vehicle Control/Dispatching
CDL/N-RV = CDL/Non-Revenue Vehicle
ASP = Armed Security Personnel

## Return to Duty Tests, Positives, and Refusals by Employee Category

| Drugs | | | | | |
|---|---|---|---|---|---|
| | RVO | RV&EM | RVC/D | CDL/N-RV | ASP |
| Testing Events | 934 | 248 | 51 | 43 | 7 |
| Refusals + Positives | 27 | 7 | 0 | 2 | 0 |
| Positives | 22 | 6 | 0 | 0 | 0 |
| Total Refusals | 5 | 1 | 0 | 2 | 0 |
| Refusal to take test | 4 | 1 | 0 | 0 | 0 |
| Shy Bladder | 0 | 0 | 0 | 2 | 0 |
| Adulterated | 0 | 0 | 0 | 0 | 0 |
| Substituted | 1 | 0 | 0 | 0 | 0 |
| Refusal Rate | 0.535 | 0.403 | 0 | 4.651 | 0 |

| Alcohol | | | | | |
|---|---|---|---|---|---|
| | RVO | RV&EM | RVC/D | CDL/N-RV | ASP |
| Testing Events | 494 | 167 | 20 | 26 | 6 |
| Refusals + Positives | 4 | 0 | 0 | 0 | 0 |
| Positives | 3 | 0 | 0 | 0 | 0 |
| Total Refusals | 1 | 0 | 0 | 0 | 0 |
| Refusal to take test | 1 | 0 | 0 | 0 | 0 |
| Shy Lung | 0 | 0 | 0 | 0 | 0 |
| Refusal Rate | 0.202 | 0 | 0 | 0 | 0 |

The rates in the preceding graph are subdivided by employer type and by employer size, respectively, in the two graphs below. The tables on the next page provide the statistical basis for the rates. *The graphs below do not contain columns for employee categories that show a rate of "0" in the preceding graph.* Some of the rates in each graph are presented on a separate scale because their sample sizes are too small to be representative of their populations. *The graph at far right contains alcohol rate columns for only large employers because no positive return to duty alcohol tests were reported by small or rural employers in 2003.*

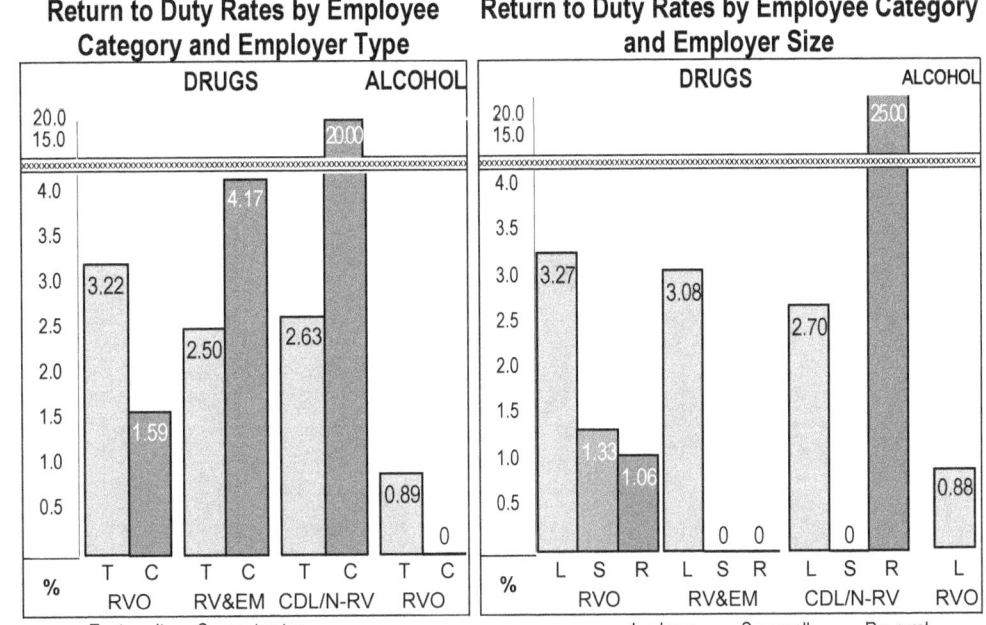

**Return to Duty Rates by Employee Category and Employer Type**

T = transit      C = contractor

**Return to Duty Rates by Employee Category and Employer Size**

L = large      S = small      R = rural

RVO = Revenue Vehicle Operation    RV&EM = Revenue Vehicle & Equipment Maintenance    CDL/N-RV = CDL/Non-Revenue Vehicle

## Return to Duty Tests, Positives, and Refusals by Employee Category and Employer Type

| Drugs | | | | | | | | | | |
|---|---|---|---|---|---|---|---|---|---|---|
| | RVO | | RV&EM | | RVC/D | | CDL/N-RV | | ASP | |
| | Transit | Contractor | Transit | Contractor | Transit | Contractor | Transit | Contractor | Transit | Contractor |
| Testing Events | 745 | 189 | 200 | 48 | 38 | 13 | 38 | 5 | 6 | 1 |
| Refusals + Positives | 24 | 3 | 5 | 2 | 0 | 0 | 1 | 1 | 0 | 0 |
| Positives | 20 | 2 | 4 | 2 | 0 | 0 | 0 | 0 | 0 | 0 |
| Total Refusals | 4 | 1 | 1 | 0 | 0 | 0 | 1 | 1 | 0 | 0 |
| Refusal to take test | 3 | 1 | 1 | 0 | 0 | 0 | 0 | 0 | 0 | 0 |
| Shy Bladder | 0 | 0 | 0 | 0 | 0 | 0 | 1 | 1 | 0 | 0 |
| Adulterated | 0 | 0 | 0 | 0 | 0 | 0 | 0 | 0 | 0 | 0 |
| Substituted | 1 | 0 | 0 | 0 | 0 | 0 | 0 | 0 | 0 | 0 |
| Refusal Rate | 0.537 | 0.529 | 0. 500 | 0 | 0 | 0 | 2.632 | 20.000 | 0 | 0 |

| Alcohol | | | | | | | | | | |
|---|---|---|---|---|---|---|---|---|---|---|
| | RVO | | RV&EM | | RVC/D | | CDL/N-RV | | ASP | |
| | Transit | Contractor | Transit | Contractor | Transit | Contractor | Transit | Contractor | Transit | Contractor |
| Testing Events | 448 | 46 | 143 | 24 | 19 | 1 | 26 | 0 | 6 | 0 |
| Refusals + Positives | 4 | 0 | 0 | 0 | 0 | 0 | 0 | 0 | 0 | 0 |
| Positives | 3 | 0 | 0 | 0 | 0 | 0 | 0 | 0 | 0 | 0 |
| Total Refusals | 1 | 0 | 0 | 0 | 0 | 0 | 0 | 0 | 0 | 0 |
| Refusal to take test | 1 | 0 | 0 | 0 | 0 | 0 | 0 | 0 | 0 | 0 |
| Shy Lung | 0 | 0 | 0 | 0 | 0 | 0 | 0 | 0 | 0 | 0 |
| Refusal Rate | 0.223 | 0 | 0 | 0 | 0 | 0 | 0 | 0 | 0 | 0 |

RVO = Revenue Vehicle Operation
RV&EM = Revenue Vehicle and Equipment Maintenance
RVC/D = Revenue Vehicle Control/Dispatching
CDL/N-RV = CDL/Non-Revenue Vehicle
ASP = Armed Security Personnel

## Return to Duty Tests, Positives, and Refusals by Employee Category and Employer Size

| Drugs | | | | | | | | | | | | | | | |
|---|---|---|---|---|---|---|---|---|---|---|---|---|---|---|---|
| | RVO | | | RV&EM | | | RVC/D | | | CDL/N-RV | | | ASP | | |
| | Large | Small | Rural | Large | Small | Rural | Large | Small | Rural | Large | Small | Rural | Large | Small | Rural |
| Testing Events | 765 | 75 | 94 | 227 | 13 | 8 | 40 | 7 | 4 | 37 | 2 | 4 | 5 | 2 | 0 |
| Refusals + Positives | 25 | 1 | 1 | 7 | 0 | 0 | 0 | 0 | 0 | 1 | 0 | 1 | 0 | 0 | 0 |
| Positives | 20 | 1 | 1 | 6 | 0 | 0 | 0 | 0 | 0 | 0 | 0 | 0 | 0 | 0 | 0 |
| Total Refusals | 5 | 0 | 0 | 1 | 0 | 0 | 0 | 0 | 0 | 1 | 0 | 1 | 0 | 0 | 0 |
| Refusal to take test | 4 | 0 | 0 | 1 | 0 | 0 | 0 | 0 | 0 | 0 | 0 | 0 | 0 | 0 | 0 |
| Shy Bladder | 0 | 0 | 0 | 0 | 0 | 0 | 0 | 0 | 0 | 1 | 0 | 1 | 0 | 0 | 0 |
| Adulterated | 0 | 0 | 0 | 0 | 0 | 0 | 0 | 0 | 0 | 0 | 0 | 0 | 0 | 0 | 0 |
| Substituted | 1 | 0 | 0 | 0 | 0 | 0 | 0 | 0 | 0 | 0 | 0 | 0 | 0 | 0 | 0 |
| Refusal Rate | 0.654 | 0 | 0 | 0.441 | 0 | 0 | 0 | 0 | 0 | 2.703 | 0 | 25.00 | 0 | 0 | 0 |

| Alcohol | | | | | | | | | | | | | | | |
|---|---|---|---|---|---|---|---|---|---|---|---|---|---|---|---|
| | RVO | | | RV&EM | | | RVC/D | | | CDL/N-RV | | | ASP | | |
| | Large | Small | Rural | Large | Small | Rural | Large | Small | Rural | Large | Small | Rural | Large | Small | Rural |
| Testing Events | 454 | 24 | 16 | 161 | 5 | 1 | 14 | 3 | 3 | 25 | 0 | 1 | 4 | 2 | 0 |
| Refusals + Positives | 4 | 0 | 0 | 0 | 0 | 0 | 0 | 0 | 0 | 0 | 0 | 0 | 0 | 0 | 0 |
| Positives | 3 | 0 | 0 | 0 | 0 | 0 | 0 | 0 | 0 | 0 | 0 | 0 | 0 | 0 | 0 |
| Total Refusals | 1 | 0 | 0 | 0 | 0 | 0 | 0 | 0 | 0 | 0 | 0 | 0 | 0 | 0 | 0 |
| Refusal to take test | 1 | 0 | 0 | 0 | 0 | 0 | 0 | 0 | 0 | 0 | 0 | 0 | 0 | 0 | 0 |
| Shy Lung | 0 | 0 | 0 | 0 | 0 | 0 | 0 | 0 | 0 | 0 | 0 | 0 | 0 | 0 | 0 |
| Refusal Rate | 0.220 | 0 | 0 | 0 | 0 | 0 | 0 | 0 | 0 | 0 | 0 | 0 | 0 | 0 | 0 |

RVO = Revenue Vehicle Operation
RV&EM = Revenue Vehicle and Equipment Maintenance
RVC/D = Revenue Vehicle Control/Dispatching
CDL/N-RV = CDL/Non-Revenue Vehicle
ASP = Armed Security Personnel

### 5.1.3 Return to Duty Test Data by FTA Region

The following map shows the rates for return to duty drug tests for each of FTA's ten regions. The shading variations enable quick comparison. The exact rates are also included. The statistical basis for those rates is provided in the accompanying table. The total number of refusals by FTA Region listed in that table is subdivided by the individual types of refusals in the table that follows the map. That table also includes the overall return to duty drug test refusal rates by FTA region.

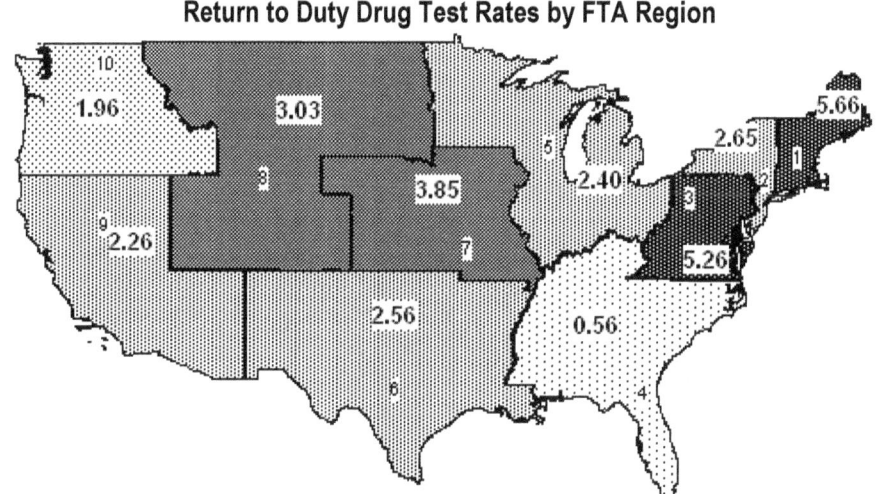

**Return to Duty Drug Test Rates by FTA Region**

**Return to Duty Drug Tests, Positives, and Refusals by FTA Region**

| Region | Testing Events | Positives | Refusals |
|--------|---------------|-----------|----------|
| 1 | 53 | 3 | 0 |
| 2 | 226 | 6 | 0 |
| 3 | 209 | 5 | 6 |
| 4 | 178 | 1 | 0 |
| 5 | 208 | 5 | 0 |
| 6 | 78 | 2 | 0 |
| 7 | 26 | 1 | 0 |
| 8 | 33 | 1 | 0 |
| 9 | 221 | 3 | 2 |
| 10 | 51 | 1 | 0 |

**Data on Return to Duty Drug Test Refusal Types by FTA Region**

| Region | 1 | 2 | 3 | 4 | 5 | 6 | 7 | 8 | 9 | 10 |
|--------|---|---|---|---|---|---|---|---|---|----|
| Refusal to take test | 0 | 0 | 3 | 0 | 0 | 0 | 0 | 0 | 2 | 0 |
| Shy Bladder | 0 | 0 | 2 | 0 | 0 | 0 | 0 | 0 | 0 | 0 |
| Adulterated | 0 | 0 | 0 | 0 | 0 | 0 | 0 | 0 | 0 | 0 |
| Substituted | 0 | 0 | 1 | 0 | 0 | 0 | 0 | 0 | 0 | 0 |
| Overall Refusal Rate | 0 | 0 | 2.871 | 0 | 0 | 0 | 0 | 0 | 0.905 | 0 |

Because only three return to duty alcohol positives and one refusal were reported in 2003, the alcohol rates for each region appear in a table, along with the statistical basis for those rates.

**Return to Duty Alcohol Data by FTA Region**

| Region | 1 | 2 | 3 | 4 | 5 | 6 | 7 | 8 | 9 | 10 |
|--------|---|---|---|---|---|---|---|---|---|----|
| Rate | 0 | 0 | 1.17 | 0 | 0 | 2.50 | 0 | 0 | 0 | 5.88 |
| Testing Events | 24 | 150 | 171 | 75 | 83 | 40 | 14 | 11 | 128 | 17 |
| Refusals + Positives | 0 | 0 | 2 | 0 | 0 | 1 | 0 | 0 | 0 | 1 |
| Positives | 0 | 0 | 1 | 0 | 0 | 1 | 0 | 0 | 0 | 1 |
| Total Refusals | 0 | 0 | 1 | 0 | 0 | 0 | 0 | 0 | 0 | 0 |
| Refusal to take test | 0 | 0 | 1 | 0 | 0 | 0 | 0 | 0 | 0 | 0 |
| Shy Lung | 0 | 0 | 0 | 0 | 0 | 0 | 0 | 0 | 0 | 0 |
| Refusal Rate | 0 | 0 | 0.585 | 0 | 0 | 0 | 0 | 0 | 0 | 0 |

## 5.1.4 Return to Duty Test Data by Type of Drug

The table at immediate right shows the number of drug testing events and the number and percent that were verified positive for each drug type. The table at far right shows the percentage by drug type of the total drug type detections. These data are subdivided by employer type, by employer size, and by employee category in the tables below.

**Return to Duty Tests, Positives, and Rates by Drug Type**

| 1,283 Testing Events | Positives | Percent |
|---|---|---|
| Marijuana | 18 | 1.40 |
| Cocaine | 8 | 0.62 |
| PCP | 0 | 0 |
| Opiates | 1 | 0.08 |
| Amphetamines | 0 | 0 |

**Percentage by Drug Type for Return to Duty Positives**

| | |
|---|---|
| Marijuana | 66.7 |
| Cocaine | 29.6 |
| PCP | 0 |
| Opiates | 3.7 |
| Amphetamines | 0 |

**Return to Duty Tests, Positives, and Rates by Employer Type and Drug Type**

| | Transit | | Contractor | |
|---|---|---|---|---|
| Testing Events | 1,027 | | 256 | |
| | Positives | Percent | Positives | Percent |
| Marijuana | 16 | 1.56 | 2 | 0.78 |
| Cocaine | 6 | 0.58 | 2 | 0.78 |
| PCP | 0 | 0 | 0 | 0 |
| Opiates | 1 | 0.10 | 0 | 0 |
| Amphetamines | 0 | 0 | 0 | 0 |

**Percentage by Employer Type and Drug Type for Return to Duty Positives**

| | Transit | Contractor |
|---|---|---|
| Marijuana | 69.6 | 50.0 |
| Cocaine | 26.1 | 50.0 |
| PCP | 0 | 0 |
| Opiates | 4.3 | 0 |
| Amphetamines | 0 | 0 |

**Return to Duty Tests, Positives, and Rates by Employer Size and Drug Type**

| | Large | | Small | | Rural | |
|---|---|---|---|---|---|---|
| Testing Events | 1,074 | | 99 | | 110 | |
| | Positives | Percent | Positives | Percent | Positives | Percent |
| Marijuana | 16 | 1.49 | 1 | 1.01 | 1 | 0.91 |
| Cocaine | 8 | 0.74 | 0 | 0 | 0 | 0 |
| PCP | 0 | 0 | 0 | 0 | 0 | 0 |
| Opiates | 1 | 0.09 | 0 | 0 | 0 | 0 |
| Amphetamines | 0 | 0.00 | 0 | 0 | 0 | 0 |

**Percentage by Employer Size and Drug Type for Return to Duty Positives**

| | Large | Small | Rural |
|---|---|---|---|
| Marijuana | 64.0 | 100 | 100 |
| Cocaine | 32.0 | 0 | 0 |
| PCP | 0 | 0 | 0 |
| Opiates | 4.0 | 0 | 0 |
| Amphetamines | 0 | 0 | 0 |

**Return to Duty Tests, Positives, and Rates by Employee Category and Drug Type**

| | RVO | | RV&EM | | RVC/D | | CDL/N-RV | | ASP | |
|---|---|---|---|---|---|---|---|---|---|---|
| Testing Events | 934 | | 248 | | 51 | | 43 | | 7 | |
| | Positives | Percent | Positives | Percent | Positives | Percent | Positives | Percent | Positives | Percent |
| Marijuana | 15 | 1.61 | 3 | 1.21 | 0 | 0 | 0 | 0 | 0 | 0 |
| Cocaine | 5 | 0.54 | 3 | 1.21 | 0 | 0 | 0 | 0 | 0 | 0 |
| PCP | 0 | 0 | 0 | 0 | 0 | 0 | 0 | 0 | 0 | 0 |
| Opiates | 1 | 0.11 | 0 | 0 | 0 | 0 | 0 | 0 | 0 | 0 |
| Amphetamines | 0 | 0 | 0 | 0 | 0 | 0 | 0 | 0 | 0 | 0 |

**Percentage by Employee Category and Drug Type for Return to Duty Positives**

| | RVO | RV&EM | RVC/D | CDL/N-RV | ASP |
|---|---|---|---|---|---|
| M | 71.4 | 50.0 | 0 | 0 | 0 |
| C | 23.8 | 50.0 | 0 | 0 | 0 |
| P | 0 | 0 | 0 | 0 | 0 |
| O | 4.8 | 0 | 0 | 0 | 0 |
| A | 0 | 0 | 0 | 0 | 0 |

RVO = Revenue Vehicle Operation          RV&EM = Revenue Vehicle and Equipment Maintenance
RVC/D = Revenue Vehicle Control/Dispatching          CDL/N-RV = CDL/Non-Revenue Vehicle          ASP = Armed Security Personnel
M = Marijuana          C = Cocaine          P = Phencyclidine (PCP)          O = Opiates          A = Amphetamines

## 5.2 Follow-Up Test Data

The combined percentage of positive tests plus test refusals for follow-up drug tests and alcohol tests are shown in the graph at right. The statistical basis for those rates is provided in the table next to the graph. The rates are subdivided by employer type and size, employee category, FTA region, and type of drug later in this section.

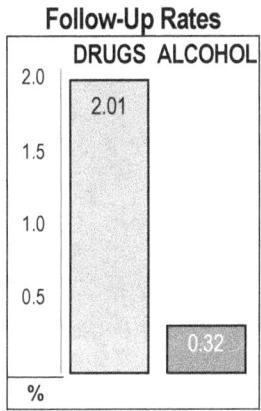

Follow-Up Rates

| | Drugs | Alcohol |
|---|---|---|
| **Follow-Up Tests, Positives, and Refusals** | | |
| Testing Events | 7,980 | 5,950 |
| Refusals + Positives | 160 | 19 |
| Positives | 149 | 17 |
| Total Refusals | 11 | 2 |
| Refusal to take test | 9 | 2 |
| Shy Bladder/ Lung | 0 | 0 |
| Adulterated | 1 | N.A. |
| Substituted | 1 | N.A. |
| Refusal Rate | 0.138 | 0.034 |

### 5.2.1 Follow-Up Test Data by Employer Type and Size

The rates in the preceding graph are subdivided by employer type, by employer size, and by employer size and type, respectively, in the following three graphs. Two of the rates in the graph at right are presented on a separate scale because their sample sizes are too small to be representative of their populations. The tables on the next page provide the statistical basis for the rates.

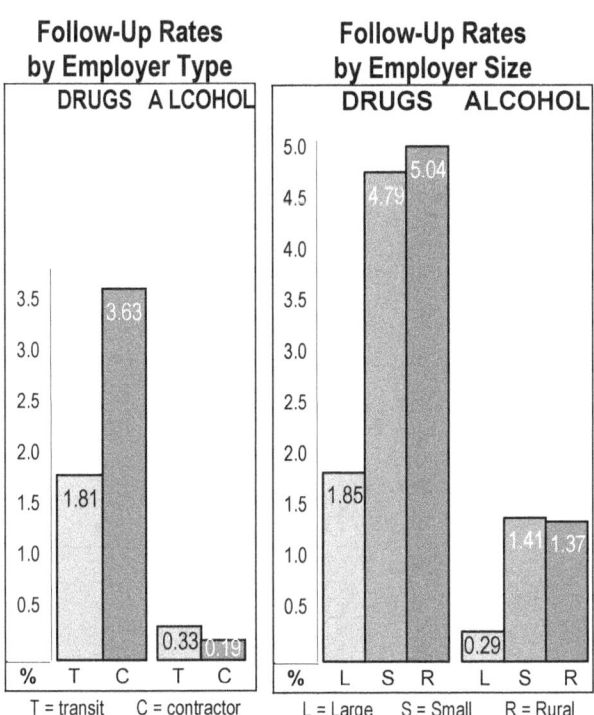

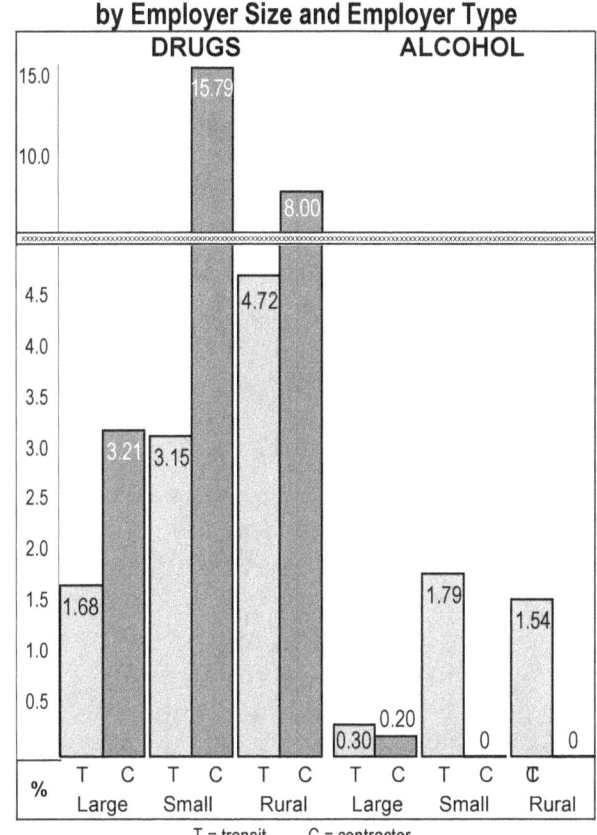

**Follow-Up Tests, Positives, and Refusals by Employer Type**

| | Drugs | | Alcohol | |
|---|---|---|---|---|
| | Transit | Contractor | Transit | Contractor |
| Testing Events | 7,126 | 854 | 5,428 | 522 |
| Refusals + Positives | 129 | 31 | 18 | 1 |
| Positives | 122 | 27 | 16 | 1 |
| Total Refusals | 7 | 4 | 2 | 0 |
|   Refusal to take test | 6 | 3 | 2 | 0 |
|   Shy Bladder/Lung | 0 | 0 | 0 | 0 |
|   Adulterated | 0 | 1 | N. A. | N. A. |
|   Substituted | 1 | 0 | N. A. | N. A. |
| Refusal Rate | 0.098 | 0.468 | 0.037 | 0 |

**Follow-Up Tests, Positives, and Refusals by Employer Size**

| | Drugs | | | Alcohol | | |
|---|---|---|---|---|---|---|
| | Large | Small | Rural | Large | Small | Rural |
| Testing Events | 7,576 | 146 | 258 | 5,806 | 71 | 73 |
| Refusals + Positives | 140 | 7 | 13 | 17 | 1 | 1 |
| Positives | 130 | 6 | 13 | 15 | 1 | 1 |
| Total Refusals | 10 | 1 | 0 | 2 | 0 | 0 |
|   Refusal to take test | 8 | 1 | 0 | 2 | 0 | 0 |
|   Shy Bladder/Lung | 0 | 0 | 0 | 0 | 0 | 0 |
|   Adulterated | 1 | 0 | 0 | N. A. | N. A. | N. A. |
|   Substituted | 1 | 0 | 0 | N. A. | N. A. | N. A. |
| Refusal Rate | 0.132 | 0.685 | 0 | 0.034 | 0 | 0 |

**Follow-Up Tests, Positives, and Refusals by Employer Size and Employer Type**

| | Drugs | | | | | | Alcohol | | | | | |
|---|---|---|---|---|---|---|---|---|---|---|---|---|
| | Large | | Small | | Rural | | Large | | Small | | Rural | |
| | Transit | Contractor | Transit | Contractor | Transit | Contractor | Transit | Contractor | Transit | Contractor | Transit | Contractor |
| Testing Events | 6,766 | 810 | 127 | 19 | 233 | 25 | 5,307 | 499 | 56 | 15 | 65 | 8 |
| Refusals + Positives | 114 | 26 | 4 | 3 | 11 | 2 | 16 | 1 | 1 | 0 | 1 | 0 |
| Positives | 108 | 22 | 3 | 3 | 11 | 2 | 14 | 1 | 1 | 0 | 1 | 0 |
| Total Refusals | 6 | 4 | 1 | 0 | 0 | 0 | 2 | 0 | 0 | 0 | 0 | 0 |
|   Refusal to take test | 5 | 3 | 1 | 0 | 0 | 0 | 2 | 0 | 0 | 0 | 0 | 0 |
|   Shy Bladder/Lung | 0 | 0 | 0 | 0 | 0 | 0 | 0 | 0 | 0 | 0 | 0 | 0 |
|   Adulterated | 0 | 1 | 0 | 0 | 0 | 0 | N. A. | N. A. | N. A. | N. A. | N. A. | N. A. |
|   Substituted | 1 | 0 | 0 | 0 | 0 | 0 | N. A. | N. A. | N. A. | N. A. | N. A. | N. A. |
| Refusal Rate | 0.089 | 0.494 | 0.787 | 0 | 0 | 0 | 0.038 | 0 | 0 | 0 | 0 | 0 |

## 5.2.2  Follow-Up Test Data by Employee Category

The graph at right shows the rates for follow-up drug tests and alcohol tests by employee category.  The table on the next page provides the statistical basis for the rates.  These data are further subdivided by employer type and employer size in the subsequent graphs and tables.  *The graphs subdivided by employer type and employer size do not contain columns for employee categories that show a rate of "0" in the graph at right.*  Three of the drug rates and one of the alcohol rates in the employer size graph are presented on a separate scale because their sample sizes are too small to be representative of their populations.

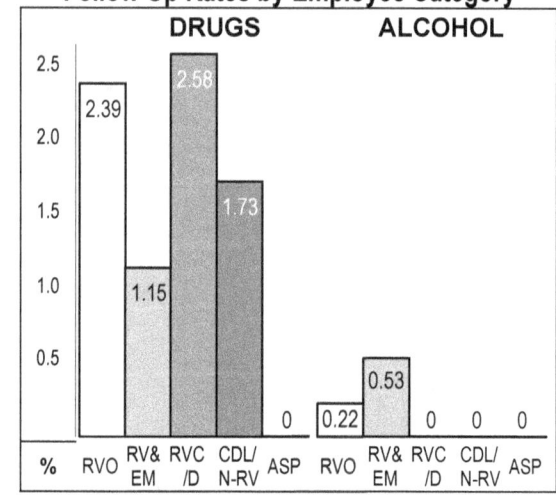

**Follow-Up Rates by Employee Category**

RVO = Revenue Vehicle Operation
RV&EM = Revenue Vehicle and Equipment Maintenance
RVC/D = Revenue Vehicle Control/Dispatching
CDL/N-RV = CDL/Non-Revenue Vehicle
ASP = Armed Security Personnel

## Follow-Up Tests, Positives, and Refusals by Employee Category

| | Drugs | | | | | Alcohol | | | | |
|---|---|---|---|---|---|---|---|---|---|---|
| | RVO | RV&EM | RVC/D | CDL/N-RV | ASP | RVO | RV&EM | RVC/D | CDL/N-RV | ASP |
| Testing Events | 5,107 | 2,357 | 271 | 231 | 14 | 3,617 | 2,058 | 161 | 114 | 0 |
| Refusals + Positives | 122 | 27 | 7 | 4 | 0 | 8 | 11 | 0 | 0 | 0 |
| Positives | 114 | 25 | 6 | 4 | 0 | 7 | 10 | 0 | 0 | 0 |
| Total Refusals | 8 | 2 | 1 | 0 | 0 | 1 | 1 | 0 | 0 | 0 |
| Refusal to take test | 6 | 2 | 1 | 0 | 0 | 1 | 1 | 0 | 0 | 0 |
| Shy Bladder | 0 | 0 | 0 | 0 | 0 | 0 | 0 | 0 | 0 | 0 |
| Adulterated | 1 | 0 | 0 | 0 | 0 | N. A. | N. A. | N. A. | N. A. | N. A. |
| Substituted | 1 | 0 | 0 | 0 | 0 | N. A. | N. A. | N. A. | N. A. | N. A. |
| Refusal Rate | 0.157 | 0.085 | 0.369 | 0 | 0 | 0.028 | 0.049 | 0 | 0 | 0 |

RVO = Revenue Vehicle Operation          RV&EM = Revenue Vehicle and Equipment Maintenance
RVC/D = Revenue Vehicle Control/Dispatching          CDL/N-RV = CDL/Non-Revenue Vehicle          ASP = Armed Security Personnel

## Follow-Up Rates by Employee Category and Employer Type

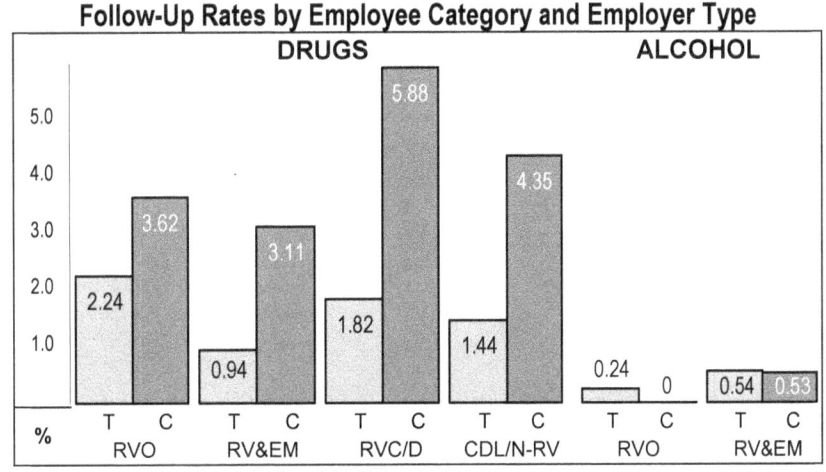

T = transit          C = contractor

RVO = Revenue Vehicle Operation          RV&EM = Revenue Vehicle and Equipment  Maintenance
RVC/D = Revenue Vehicle Control/Dispatching          CDL/N-RV = CDL/Non-Revenue Vehicle

## Follow-Up Rates by Employee Category and Employer Size

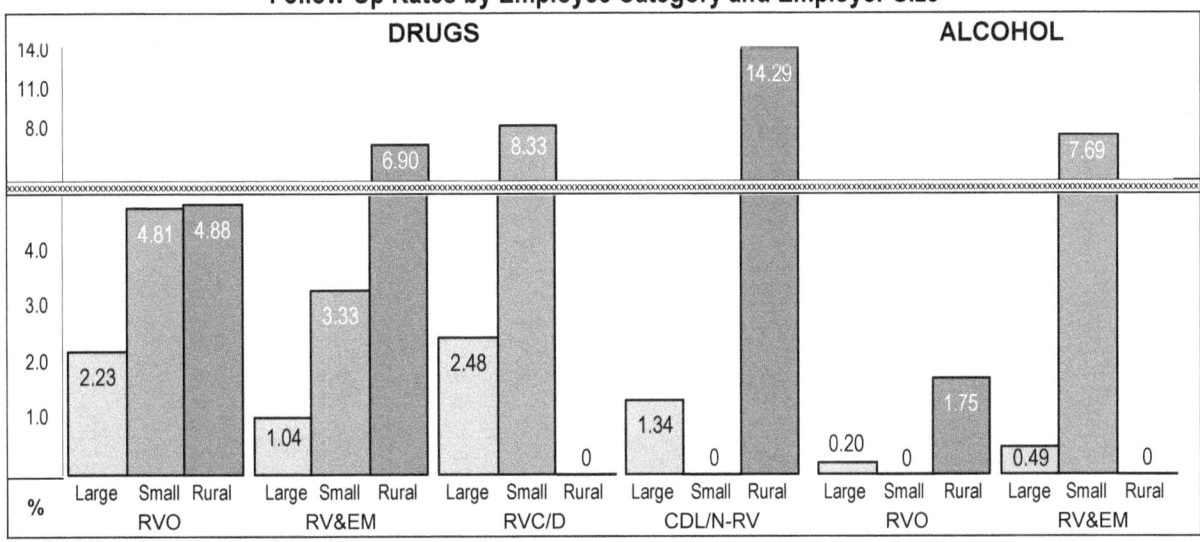

RVO = Revenue Vehicle Operation          RV&EM = Revenue Vehicle and Equipment  Maintenance
RVC/D = Revenue Vehicle Control/Dispatching          CDL/N-RV = CDL/Non-Revenue Vehicle

## Follow-Up Tests, Positives, and Refusals by Employee Category and Employer Type

### Drugs

| | RVO | | RV&EM | | RVC/D | | CDL/N-RV | | ASP | |
|---|---|---|---|---|---|---|---|---|---|---|
| | Transit | Contractor | Transit | Contractor | Transit | Contractor | Transit | Contractor | Transit | Contractor |
| Testing Events | 4,554 | 553 | 2,132 | 225 | 220 | 51 | 208 | 23 | 12 | 2 |
| Refusals + Positives | 102 | 20 | 20 | 7 | 4 | 3 | 3 | 1 | 0 | 0 |
| Positives | 97 | 17 | 18 | 7 | 4 | 2 | 3 | 1 | 0 | 0 |
| Total Refusals | 5 | 3 | 2 | 0 | 0 | 1 | 0 | 0 | 0 | 0 |
| Refusal to take test | 4 | 2 | 2 | 0 | 0 | 1 | 0 | 0 | 0 | 0 |
| Shy Bladder | 0 | 0 | 0 | 0 | 0 | 0 | 0 | 0 | 0 | 0 |
| Adulterated | 0 | 1 | 0 | 0 | 0 | 0 | 0 | 0 | 0 | 0 |
| Substituted | 1 | 0 | 0 | 0 | 0 | 0 | 0 | 0 | 0 | 0 |
| Refusal Rate | 0.110 | 0.542 | 0.094 | 0 | 0 | 0.1961 | 0 | 0 | 0 | 0 |

### Alcohol

| | RVO | | RV&EM | | RVC/D | | CDL/N-RV | | ASP | |
|---|---|---|---|---|---|---|---|---|---|---|
| | Transit | Contractor | Transit | Contractor | Transit | Contractor | Transit | Contractor | Transit | Contractor |
| Testing Events | 3,318 | 299 | 1,868 | 190 | 139 | 22 | 103 | 11 | 0 | 0 |
| Refusals + Positives | 8 | 0 | 10 | 1 | 0 | 0 | 0 | 0 | 0 | 0 |
| Positives | 7 | 0 | 9 | 1 | 0 | 0 | 0 | 0 | 0 | 0 |
| Total Refusals | 1 | 0 | 1 | 0 | 0 | 0 | 0 | 0 | 0 | 0 |
| Refusal to take test | 1 | 0 | 1 | 0 | 0 | 0 | 0 | 0 | 0 | 0 |
| Shy Lung | 0 | 0 | 0 | 0 | 0 | 0 | 0 | 0 | 0 | 0 |
| Refusal Rate | 0.030 | 0 | 0.054 | 0 | 0 | 0 | 0 | 0 | 0 | 0 |

RVO = Revenue Vehicle Operation    RV&EM = Revenue Vehicle and Equipment Maintenance
RVC/D = Revenue Vehicle Control/Dispatching    CDL/N-RV = CDL/Non-Revenue Vehicle    ASP = Armed Security Personnel

## Follow-Up Tests, Positives, and Refusals by Employee Category and Employer Size

### Drugs

| | RVO | | | RV&EM | | | RVC/D | | | CDL/N-RV | | | ASP | | |
|---|---|---|---|---|---|---|---|---|---|---|---|---|---|---|---|
| | Large | Small | Rural | Large | Small | Rural | Large | Small | Rural | Large | Small | Rural | Large | Small | Rural |
| Testing Events | 4,798 | 104 | 205 | 2,298 | 30 | 29 | 242 | 12 | 17 | 224 | 0 | 7 | 14 | 0 | 0 |
| Refusals + Positives | 107 | 5 | 10 | 24 | 1 | 2 | 6 | 1 | 0 | 3 | 0 | 1 | 0 | 0 | 0 |
| Positives | 100 | 4 | 10 | 22 | 1 | 2 | 5 | 1 | 0 | 3 | 0 | 1 | 0 | 0 | 0 |
| Total Refusals | 7 | 1 | 0 | 2 | 0 | 0 | 1 | 0 | 0 | 0 | 0 | 0 | 0 | 0 | 0 |
| Refusal to take test | 5 | 1 | 0 | 2 | 0 | 0 | 1 | 0 | 0 | 0 | 0 | 0 | 0 | 0 | 0 |
| Shy Bladder | 0 | 0 | 0 | 0 | 0 | 0 | 0 | 0 | 0 | 0 | 0 | 0 | 0 | 0 | 0 |
| Adulterated | 1 | 0 | 0 | 0 | 0 | 0 | 0 | 0 | 0 | 0 | 0 | 0 | 0 | 0 | 0 |
| Substituted | 1 | 0 | 0 | 0 | 0 | 0 | 0 | 0 | 0 | 0 | 0 | 0 | 0 | 0 | 0 |
| Refusal Rate | 0.146 | 0.962 | 0 | 0.087 | 0 | 0 | 0.413 | 0 | 0 | 0 | 0 | 0 | 0 | 0 | 0 |

### Alcohol

| | RVO | | | RV&EM | | | RVC/D | | | CDL/N-RV | | | ASP | | |
|---|---|---|---|---|---|---|---|---|---|---|---|---|---|---|---|
| | Large | Small | Rural | Large | Small | Rural | Large | Small | Rural | Large | Small | Rural | Large | Small | Rural |
| Testing Events | 3,502 | 58 | 57 | 2,037 | 13 | 8 | 154 | 0 | 7 | 113 | 0 | 1 | 0 | 0 | 0 |
| Refusals + Positives | 7 | 0 | 1 | 10 | 1 | 0 | 0 | 0 | 0 | 0 | 0 | 0 | 0 | 0 | 0 |
| Positives | 6 | 0 | 1 | 9 | 1 | 0 | 0 | 0 | 0 | 0 | 0 | 0 | 0 | 0 | 0 |
| Total Refusals | 1 | 0 | 0 | 1 | 0 | 0 | 0 | 0 | 0 | 0 | 0 | 0 | 0 | 0 | 0 |
| Refusal to take test | 1 | 0 | 0 | 1 | 0 | 0 | 0 | 0 | 0 | 0 | 0 | 0 | 0 | 0 | 0 |
| Shy Lung | 0 | 0 | 0 | 0 | 0 | 0 | 0 | 0 | 0 | 0 | 0 | 0 | 0 | 0 | 0 |
| Refusal Rate | 0.029 | 0 | 0 | 0.049 | 0 | 0 | 0 | 0 | 0 | 0 | 0 | 0 | 0 | 0 | 0 |

RVO = Revenue Vehicle Operation    RV&EM = Revenue Vehicle and Equipment Maintenance
RVC/D = Revenue Vehicle Control/Dispatching    CDL/N-RV = CDL/Non-Revenue Vehicle    ASP = Armed Security Personnel

### 5.2.3 Follow-Up Test Data by FTA Region

The following two maps show the rates for follow-up drug tests and alcohol tests for each of FTA's ten regions. The shading variations enable quick comparison. The exact rates are also included. The statistical basis for those rates is provided in the accompanying tables. The total number of test refusals is subdivided by the individual types of refusals in the table following the maps.

#### Follow-Up Drug Rates by FTA Region

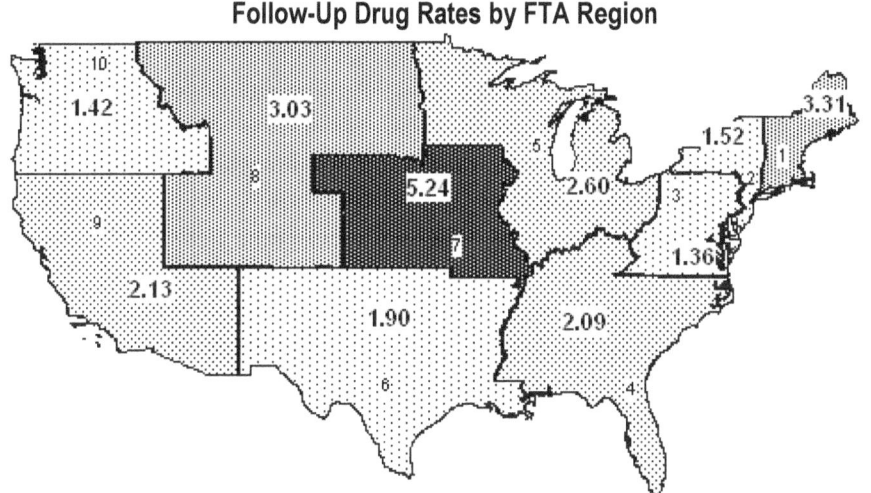

#### Follow-Up Drug Tests, Positives, and Refusals by FTA Region

| Region | Testing Events | Positives | Refusals |
|---|---|---|---|
| 1 | 302 | 10 | 0 |
| 2 | 1,904 | 26 | 3 |
| 3 | 1,474 | 17 | 3 |
| 4 | 382 | 8 | 0 |
| 5 | 1,310 | 33 | 1 |
| 6 | 316 | 6 | 0 |
| 7 | 191 | 10 | 0 |
| 8 | 198 | 4 | 2 |
| 9 | 1,409 | 28 | 2 |
| 10 | 494 | 7 | 0 |

#### Follow-Up Alcohol Rates by FTA Region

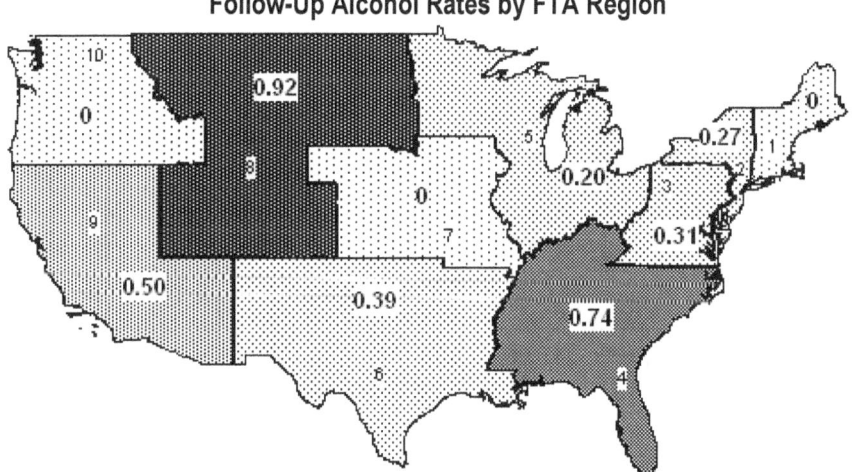

#### Follow-Up Alcohol Tests, Positives, and Refusals by FTA Region

| Region | Testing Events | Positives | Refusals |
|---|---|---|---|
| 1 | 243 | 0 | 0 |
| 2 | 1,819 | 5 | 0 |
| 3 | 1,276 | 3 | 1 |
| 4 | 136 | 1 | 0 |
| 5 | 506 | 1 | 0 |
| 6 | 259 | 1 | 0 |
| 7 | 87 | 0 | 0 |
| 8 | 109 | 1 | 0 |
| 9 | 1,203 | 5 | 1 |
| 10 | 312 | 0 | 0 |

#### Data on Return to Duty Drug Test Refusal Types by FTA Region

| Region | Drugs 1 | 2 | 3 | 4 | 5 | 6 | 7 | 8 | 9 | 10 | Alcohol 1 | 2 | 3 | 4 | 5 | 6 | 7 | 8 | 9 | 10 |
|---|---|---|---|---|---|---|---|---|---|---|---|---|---|---|---|---|---|---|---|---|
| RTT | 0 | 2 | 3 | 0 | 1 | 0 | 0 | 2 | 1 | 0 | 0 | 0 | 1 | 0 | 0 | 0 | 0 | 0 | 1 | 0 |
| SB | 0 | 0 | 0 | 0 | 0 | 0 | 0 | 0 | 0 | 0 | 0 | 0 | 0 | 0 | 0 | 0 | 0 | 0 | 0 | 0 |
| Adul | 0 | 1 | 0 | 0 | 0 | 0 | 0 | 0 | 0 | 0 | N.A. | N.A. | N.A. | N.A. | N.A. | N.A. | N.A. | N.A. | N.A. | N.A. |
| Sub | 0 | 0 | 0 | 0 | 0 | 0 | 0 | 0 | 1 | 0 | N.A. | N.A. | N.A. | N.A. | N.A. | N.A. | N.A. | N.A. | N.A. | N.A. |
| R Rate | 0 | 0.158 | 0.204 | 0 | 0.076 | 0 | 0 | 1.010 | 0.142 | 0 | 0 | 0 | 0.078 | 0 | 0 | 0 | 0 | 0 | 0.083 | 0 |

RTT = refusal to take test    SB = shy bladder    SL = shy lung    Adul = adulterated    Sub = substituted    R Rate = overall refusal rate

---

### 5.2.4 Follow-Up Test Data by Type of Drug

The two tables at right show follow-up test data for each type of drug tested for. The table at immediate right shows the number of testing events and the number and percent of those verified positive by drug type. The table at far right shows the percentage by drug type of the total drug type detections. These data are divided by employer type, employer size, and employee category in the tables that follow.

**Follow-Up Tests, Positives, and Rates by Drug Type**

| 7,980 Testing Events | Positives | Percent |
|---|---|---|
| Marijuana | 58 | 0.73 |
| Cocaine | 79 | 0.99 |
| PCP | 0 | 0 |
| Opiates | 4 | 0.05 |
| Amphetamines | 11 | 0.14 |

**Percentage by Drug Type for Follow-Up Positives**

| | |
|---|---|
| Marijuana | 38.2 |
| Cocaine | 52.0 |
| PCP | 0 |
| Opiates | 2.6 |
| Amphetamines | 7.2 |

**Follow-Up Tests, Positives, and Rates by Employer Type and Drug Type**

| | Transit | | Contractor | |
|---|---|---|---|---|
| Testing Events | 7,126 | | 854 | |
| | Positives | Percent | Positives | Percent |
| Marijuana | 47 | 0.66 | 11 | 1.30 |
| Cocaine | 68 | 0.95 | 11 | 1.30 |
| PCP | 0 | 0 | 0 | 0 |
| Opiates | 4 | 0.06 | 0 | 0 |
| Amphetamines | 8 | 0.11 | 3 | 0.35 |

**Percentage by Employer Type and Drug Type for Follow-Up Positives**

| | Transit | Contractor |
|---|---|---|
| Marijuana | 37.0 | 44.0 |
| Cocaine | 53.6 | 44.0 |
| PCP | 0 | 0 |
| Opiates | 3.1 | 0 |
| Amphetamines | 6.3 | 12.0 |

**Follow-Up Tests, Positives, and Rates by Employer Size and Drug Type**

| | Large | | Small | | Rural | |
|---|---|---|---|---|---|---|
| Testing Events | 7,576 | | 146 | | 258 | |
| | Positives | Percent | Positives | Percent | Positives | Percent |
| Marijuana | 52 | 0.69 | 3 | 2.05 | 3 | 2.05 |
| Cocaine | 68 | 0.90 | 3 | 2.05 | 8 | 5.48 |
| PCP | 0 | 0 | 0 | 0 | 0 | 0 |
| Opiates | 4 | 0.05 | 0 | 0 | 0 | 0 |
| Amphetamines | 9 | 0.12 | 0 | 0 | 2 | 0.78 |

**Percentage by Employer Size and Drug Type for Follow-Up Positives**

| | Large | Small | Rural |
|---|---|---|---|
| Marijuana | 39.1 | 50.0 | 23.1 |
| Cocaine | 51.1 | 50.0 | 61.5 |
| PCP | 0 | 0 | 0 |
| Opiates | 3.0 | 0 | 0 |
| Amphetamines | 6.8 | 0 | 15.4 |

**Follow-Up Tests, Positives, and Rates by Employee Category and Drug Type**

| | RVO | | RV&EM | | RVC/D | | CDL/N-RV | | ASP | |
|---|---|---|---|---|---|---|---|---|---|---|
| Testing Events | 5,107 | | 2,357 | | 271 | | 231 | | 14 | |
| | Positives | Percent | Positives | Percent | Positives | Percent | Positives | Percent | Positives | Percent |
| Marijuana | 41 | 0.80 | 11 | 0.47 | 3 | 1.11 | 3 | 1.30 | 0 | 0 |
| Cocaine | 66 | 1.29 | 11 | 0 | 2 | 0.74 | 0 | 0 | 0 | 0 |
| PCP | 0 | 0 | 0 | 0 | 0 | 0 | 0 | 0 | 0 | 0 |
| Opiates | 3 | 0.06 | 1 | 0.04 | 0 | 0 | 0 | 0 | 0 | 0 |
| Amphetamines | 7 | 0.14 | 4 | 0.17 | 0 | 0 | 0 | 0 | 0 | 0 |

**Percentage by Employee Category and Drug Type for Follow-Up Positives**

| | RVO | RV&EM | RVC/D | CDL/N-RV | ASP |
|---|---|---|---|---|---|
| M | 35.0 | 40.7 | 60.0 | 100 | 0 |
| C | 56.4 | 40.7 | 40.0 | 0 | 0 |
| P | 0 | 0 | 0 | 0 | 0 |
| O | 2.6 | 3.7 | 0 | 0 | 0 |
| A | 6.0 | 14.8 | 0 | 0 | 0 |

RVO = Revenue Vehicle Operation    RV&EM = Revenue Vehicle and Equipment Maintenance
RVC/D = Revenue Vehicle Control/Dispatching    CDL/N-RV = CDL/Non-Revenue Vehicle    ASP = Armed Security Personnel

# Appendix A. Glossary

**Alcohol:** The intoxicating agent in beverage alcohol, ethyl alcohol, or other low molecular weight alcohols including methyl or isopropyl alcohol.

**Alcohol concentration:** The alcohol in a volume of breath expressed in terms of grams of alcohol per 210 liters of breath as indicated by a breath test using an evidential breath testing (EBT) device.

**Alcohol positive:** A confirmed specimen with a breath alcohol level of at least 0.04.

**Alcohol use:** The consumption of any beverage, mixture, or preparation, including any medication containing alcohol.

**Armed security personnel:** A safety-sensitive employee category that includes any person who provides security to protect persons or property, and any person who carries a firearm.

**Canceled or invalid test:** A drug or alcohol test that has been declared invalid by a Medical Review Officer (MRO). It is neither a positive nor a negative test.

**CDL/non-revenue vehicle:** A safety-sensitive employee category that includes any person who holds a Commercial Driver's License (CDL), performs a function requiring a CDL, and is not included in any other job category.

**Confirmed alcohol specimen (or test result):** The breath alcohol level obtained using an evidential breath testing (EBT) device. The specimen, referred to as a confirmation test, is required to be taken from any employee who completes an initial screening test producing a breath alcohol level of at least 0.02. The confirmed result is the official alcohol test result.

**Consortium:** An entity, including a group or association of employers, operators, recipients, subrecipients, or contractors, that provides drug testing services and acts on behalf of the employer.

**Contractor:** A person or organization that provides a service for a recipient, subrecipient, employer, or operator consistent with a specific understanding or arrangement. The understanding can be a written contract or an informal arrangement that reflects an ongoing relationship between the parties.

**Drug metabolite:** The specific substance produced when the human body metabolizes a prohibited drug as it passes through the body and is excreted in urine.

**Drug positive:**  See "verified positive."

**Drug type:**  A classification of the five prohibited substances that must be tested for in accordance with Part 40: marijuana, cocaine, phencyclidine (PCP), opiates, and amphetamines.

**Employee category:**  One of five classifications of safety-sensitive employees defined by Part 655.  The categories are listed under "safety-sensitive employees" and each category is defined under its title.

**Employer:**  A recipient or other entity that provides mass transportation services or performs a safety-sensitive function for such recipient or other entity.  This term includes subrecipients, operators, and contractors.

**Employer size:**  A classification of employers based on the population of the primary area in which they operate: large, small, or rural.  These categories are defined under "large employers," "small employers," and "rural employers," respectively.

**Employer type:**  A classification of employers based on whether they receive funding from FTA: transit agency or contractor.  These categories are defined under their titles.

**Follow-up testing:**  Required of employees who have returned to duty in a safety-sensitive position following a verified positive drug test, a confirmed alcohol result of 0.04 or greater, a refusal to submit to a test, or any other violation of Part 40 or 655.  A minimum of six tests for the test or violation at issue (drug or alcohol) must be performed during the first 12 months after the employee returns to duty.  Testing for both drugs and alcohol is permitted.  The SAP can require that additional follow-up tests be performed, up to 5 years following return to duty.

**FTA:**  The Federal Transit Administration, an agency of the U.S. Department of Transportation (DOT).

**Large operator:**  A recipient or subrecipient primarily operating in an area with a population of 200,000 or more.

**Medical Review Officer (MRO):**  A licensed physician (Doctor of Medicine or Doctor of Osteopathy) who is responsible for receiving laboratory results generated by an employer's drug testing program and who has knowledge of substance abuse disorders and appropriate medical training to interpret and evaluate a person's positive test result together with appropriate medical history and any other relevant biomedical information.

**Part 40:** US DOT's testing regulation titled *Procedures for Transportation Workplace Drug and Alcohol Testing Programs*, which was enacted in 1994, revised in 2000, and amended in 2003.

**Part 655:** FTA's testing regulation titled *Prevention of Alcohol Misuse and Prohibited Drug Use in Transit Operations*. In was enacted in 2001 to expand the minimum requirements of the revised Part 40 and to combine the previous FTA testing regulations enacted in 1994: Part 653, *Prevention of Prohibited Drug Use in Transit Operations*, and Part 654, *Prevention of Alcohol Misuse in Transit Operations*.

**Post-accident testing:** Required for both prohibited drugs and alcohol following a mass transit accident that meets any of three other criteria and the employee's involvement cannot be completely discounted as a contributing factor: (1) when a person suffers a bodily injury and immediately receives medical attention away from the scene, (2) when any vehicle involved in the accident incurs damage requiring it to be transported away from the scene by a tow truck or other vehicle, or (3) when the mass transit vehicle involved is a rail car, trolley car, trolley bus, or vessel and is removed from revenue service due to the accident. Employees to be tested include the vehicle operator and any other safety-sensitive employee not in the vehicle whose performance could have contributed to the accident.

**Pre-employment testing:** Required for drugs before an applicant or existing employee performs a safety-sensitive function for the first time or following an absence from safety-sensitive duties for more than 90 consecutive calendar days. Employers are not required to perform pre-employment alcohol tests, but are permitted to perform such tests under their own authority providing they are performed in accordance with the requirements of Part 40.

**Random testing:** Required for both drugs and alcohol for a certain percentage (specified by the FTA Administrator) of each employer's safety-sensitive employees each year. The tests are to be unannounced, the pattern is to unpredictable, and tests are to be performed during all days and hours that employees in the random pool perform safety-sensitive duties. Employees are selected based on a scientifically valid random-number selection method. Random testing is considered by FTA to be the most effective deterrent to drug use and alcohol misuse.

**Random testing rate:** The rate at which each employer must conduct random tests each year. The number of random drug tests must equal a percentage (specified by FTA each year) of the number of the employer's safety-sensitive employees. In 2002, the drug testing rate was 50 percent, and the alcohol testing rate was 10 percent. These rates remained the same in 2003. They can be amended (per Part 655.45) by the FTA Administrator based on the combined percentage of positive tests plus test refusals.

**Reasonable suspicion testing:** Required when an employer has reasonable suspicion that an employee has used a prohibited drug or has misused alcohol as defined in Part 40. Reasonable suspicion testing must be based on specific, contemporaneous, articulable observations made by a trained supervisor concerning the appearance, behavior, speech, or body odor of a safety-sensitive employee.

**Recipient:** An entity receiving financial assistance under Section 5307, 5309, or 5311 of the Federal Transit Act or under Section 103(e)(4) of Title 23 of the U.S. Code. A *direct recipient* receives funding directly from FTA, i.e., most large transit agencies, state governments, and metropolitan planning organizations (MPOs). A *subrecipient* receives funding from a state government or from an MPO.

**Return to duty testing:** Required before an employee is allowed to return to duty to perform a safety-sensitive function following a verified positive drug test, a confirmed alcohol result of 0.04 or greater, a refusal to submit to a test, or any other violation of Part 40 or 655. The test performed (drug or alcohol) must be the same as the test or violation at issue. Testing for both drugs and alcohol is permitted.

**Revenue vehicle and equipment maintenance:** A safety-sensitive employee category that includes any person who maintains revenue service vehicles or equipment. It also includes many maintenance contract employees who perform routine, ongoing repair or maintenance for FTA recipients and subrecipients that have employees, including supervisors, who perform or could be called upon to perform any of the FTA safety-sensitive functions. Maintenance contractors of 5311 funding recipients are not subject to the testing regulations.

**Revenue vehicle control/dispatching:** A safety-sensitive employee category that includes any person who controls the dispatch or movement of revenue service vehicles.

**Revenue vehicle operations:** A safety-sensitive employee category that includes any person who operates or works as a crewman on revenue service vehicles at any time, even if the vehicles are not in service.

**Rural operator:** A subrecipient of 5311 funding primarily operating in an area with a population of less than 50,000.

**Safety-sensitive employee:** An employee who performs any of the five safety-sensitive job functions specified in Part 40:

- Revenue vehicle operations
- Revenue vehicle and equipment maintenance
- Revenue vehicle control/dispatching
- CDL/non-revenue vehicle
- Armed security personnel

**Small operator:** A recipient or subrecipient primarily operating in an area with a population of 50,000 or greater and less than 200,000.

**Substance Abuse Professional (SAP):** A licensed physician (Doctor of Medicine or Doctor of Osteopathy), or a licensed or certified psychologist, social worker, employee assistance professional, or addiction counselor (certified by the National Association of Alcoholism and Drug Abuse Counselors Certification Commission), with knowledge of and clinical experience in the diagnosis and treatment of drug and alcohol-related disorders.

**Test refusal:** Failure to produce a required urine or breath screen or specimen in accordance with Part 40. There are four types of drug test refusals and two types of alcohol test refusals:

- Adulterated – submittal of an adulterated urine specimen
- Substituted – submittal of urine not produced at the collection site
- Shy bladder with no medical explanation – failure to provide enough urine at the collection site, and no medical reason for the failure is found by the MRO
- Other refusals to submit to drug testing – Examples include failure to report to the collection site as directed by the employer, leaving the collection site without permission, and failure to empty pockets at the collection site.
- Shy lung with no medical explanation – failure to provide enough breath at the collection site, and no medical reason for the failure is found by the MRO
- Other refusals to submit to alcohol testing – same examples as for drug tests

**Test type:** A classification of the five circumstances that safety-sensitive employees must be tested for in accordance with Part 40: random, post-accident, reasonable suspicion, pre-employment, and return to duty/follow-up (which consists of both return to duty tests and follow-up tests, in accordance with Part 655). These test types are defined under their titles.

**Testing event:** A scheduled test that is submitted to or refused by the employee and not canceled by the MRO.

**Transit agency:** The public entity responsible for providing mass transit services that receives funding from FTA, either directly from FTA or indirectly from a state government or MPO.

**Verified drug positive:** A urine specimen with a concentration above the minimum thresholds specified in Part 40 obtained during a second urine test procedure and verified by an MRO during an independent review conducted in accordance with Part 40. A second test is required for any employee who produces a positive result in the initial drug screening test. The verified result, which identifies and quantifies the presence of any of the five prohibited drugs or drug metabolites, is the official drug test result. Both the initial and second specimens must be collected in accordance with Part 40 and analyzed in a DHHS-approved laboratory.

# Appendix B. FTA Regions

The Federal Transit Administration (FTA) has ten regions, which are identified below. The data provided by these regions have facilitated the comparison of drug and alcohol test results and the identification of regional trends.

## U.S. States and Territories Reporting to the 10 FTA Regions

| Region 1 | Region 2 | Region 3 | Region 4 | Region 5 |
|---|---|---|---|---|
| Connecticut | New Jersey | Delaware | Alabama | Illinois |
| Maine | New York | District of | Florida | Indiana |
| Massachusetts | Virgin Islands | Columbia | Georgia | Michigan |
| New Hampshire | | Maryland | Kentucky | Minnesota |
| Rhode Island | | Pennsylvania | Mississippi | Ohio |
| Vermont | | Virginia | North Carolina | Wisconsin |
| | | West Virginia | Puerto Rico | |
| | | | South Carolina | |
| | | | Tennessee | |

| Region 6 | Region 7 | Region 8 | Region 9 | Region 10 |
|---|---|---|---|---|
| Arkansas | Iowa | Colorado | American Samoa | Alaska |
| Louisiana | Kansas | Montana | Arizona | Idaho |
| New Mexico | Missouri | North Dakota | California | Oregon |
| Oklahoma | Nebraska | South Dakota | Guam | Washington |
| Texas | | Utah | Hawaii | |
| | | Wyoming | Nevada | |
| | | | Northern | |
| | | | Mariana Islands | |

# Appendix C. MIS Data Collection Form

**U.S. DEPARTMENT OF TRANSPORTATION DRUG AND ALCOHOL TESTING MIS DATA COLLECTION FORM**

Calendar Year Covered by this Report: _____     OMB No 2105-0529

## I. Employer:

Company Name:_____

Doing Business As (DBA) Name (if applicable):_____

Address:_____ E-mail: _____

Name of Certifying Official: _____ Signature: _____

Telephone: (____)_____ Date Certified: _____

Prepared by (if different): _____ Telephone: (____)_____

C/TPA Name and Telephone (if applicable): _____ (____)_____

**Check the DOT agency for which you are reporting MIS data; and complete the information on that same line as appropriate**:

___ FMCSA – Motor Carrier: DOT #: _____ Owner-operator: (circle one) YES or NO   Exempt (Circle One) YES or NO

___ FAA – Aviation: Certificate # (if applicable): _____ Plan / Registration # (if applicable):_____

___ RSPA – Pipeline: (Check) Gas Gathering__ Gas Transmission__ Gas Distribution__ Transport Hazardous Liquids__ Transport Carbon Dioxide__

___ FRA – Railroad: Total Number of observed/documented Part 219 "Rule G" Observations for covered employees: _____

___ USCG – Maritime: Vessel ID # (USCG- or State-Issued): _____ (If more than one vessel, list separately.)

___ FTA – Transit

## II. Covered Employees:

**(A)** Enter Total Number Safety-Sensitive Employees In All Employee Categories: [_____]

**(B)** Enter Total Number of Employee Categories: [_____]

**(C)**

| Employee Category | Total Number of Employees in this Category | If you have multiple employee categories, complete Sections I and II (A) & (B). Take that filled-in form and make one copy for each employee category and complete Sections II (C), III, and IV for each separate employee category. |
|---|---|---|
| | | |

## III. Drug Testing Data:

| Type of Test | 1 Total Number Of Test Results [Should equal the sum of Columns 2, 3, 9, 10, 11, and 12] | 2 Verified Negative Results | 3 Verified Positive Results ~ For One Or More Drugs | 4 Positive For Marijuana | 5 Positive For Cocaine | 6 Positive For PCP | 7 Positive For Opiates | 8 Positive For Amphetamines | Refusal Results 9 Adulterated | 10 Substituted | 11 "Shy Bladder" ~ With No Medical Explanation | 12 Other Refusals To Submit To Testing | 13 Cancelled Results |
|---|---|---|---|---|---|---|---|---|---|---|---|---|---|
| Pre-Employment | | | | | | | | | | | | | |
| Random | | | | | | | | | | | | | |
| Post-Accident | | | | | | | | | | | | | |
| Reasonable Susp./Cause | | | | | | | | | | | | | |
| Return-to-Duty | | | | | | | | | | | | | |
| Follow-Up | | | | | | | | | | | | | |
| TOTAL | | | | | | | | | | | | | |

## IV. Alcohol Testing Data:

| Type of Test | 1 Total Number Of Screening Test Results [Should equal the sum of Columns 2, 3, 7, and 8] | 2 Screening Tests With Results Below 0.02 | 3 Screening Tests With Results 0.02 Or Greater | 4 Number Of Confirmation Tests Results | 5 Confirmation Tests With Results 0.02 Through 0.039 | 6 Confirmation Tests With Results 0.04 Or Greater | Refusal Results 7 "Shy Lung" ~ With No Medical Explanation | 8 Other Refusals To Submit To Testing | 9 Cancelled Results |
|---|---|---|---|---|---|---|---|---|---|
| Pre-Employment | | | | | | | | | |
| Random | | | | | | | | | |
| Post-Accident | | | | | | | | | |
| Reasonable Susp./Cause | | | | | | | | | |
| Return-to-Duty | | | | | | | | | |
| Follow-Up | | | | | | | | | |
| TOTAL | | | | | | | | | |

Title 18, USC Section 1001, makes it a criminal offense subject to a maximum fine of $10,000, or imprisonment for not more than 5 years, or both, to knowingly and willfully make or cause to be made any false or fraudulent statements of representations in any matter within the jurisdiction of any agency of the United States.

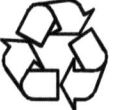

www.ingramcontent.com/pod-product-compliance
Lightning Source LLC
Chambersburg PA
CBHW080427290526
45791CB00008BA/2424